Psychiatry at a Glance

Cornelius Katona

MD, FRCPsych
Dean, Kent Institute of Medicine and Health Sciences, University of Kent
Hon. Consultant Psychiatrist, East Kent Partnership Trust

Mary Robertson

MD, MRCPCH, FRCP, FRCPsych
Emeritus Professor
Royal Free and University College Medical School
Department of Mental Health Sciences
Visiting Professor, St George's Hospital Medical School
Department of Mental Health Sciences
Hon. Consultant Psychiatrist, St George's Hospital

Third edition

Blackwell Publishing

Published by Blackwell Publishing Ltd
Blackwell Publishing, Inc., 350 Main Street, Malden, Massachusetts 02148-5020, USA
Blackwell Publishing Ltd, 9600 Garsington Road, Oxford OX4 2DQ, UK
Blackwell Publishing Asia Pty Ltd, 550 Swanston Street, Carlton, Victoria 3053, Australia

First published 1995
Second edition 2000
Reprinted 2000, 2001, 2005
Third edition 2005

Library of Congress Cataloging-in-Publication Data

Katona, C. L. E. (Cornelius L. E.), 1954–
    Psychiatry at a glance / Cornelius Katona, Mary Robertson. —3rd ed.
    p.   ;   cm.
    Includes bibliographical references and index.
    ISBN-10: 1-4051-2404-0
    ISBN-13: 978-1-4051-2404-1
1. Psychiatry.
[DNLM: 1. Mental Disorders.   2. Psychiatry.]   I. Robertson, Mary M.   II. Title.

RC454.K366   2005
616.89—dc22

                                                                    2005001829

ISBN-13: 978-1-4051-2404-1
ISBN-10: 1-4051-2404-0

A catalogue record for this title is available from the British Library

Set in 9.5 on 12pt Times New Roman PS by SNP Best-set Typesetter Ltd., Hong Kong
Printed and bound in India by Replika Press Pvt., Ltd

Commissioning Editor: Martin Sugden
Development Editor: Fiona Pattison
Production Controller: Kate Charman

For further information on Blackwell Publishing, visit our website:
http://www.blackwellpublishing.com

The publisher's policy is to use permanent paper from mills that operate a sustainable forestry policy, and
which has been manufactured from pulp processed using acid-free and elementary chlorine-free practices.
Furthermore, the publisher ensures that the text paper and cover board used have met acceptable
environmental accreditation standards.

Psychiatry at a Glance

Contents

Introduction to the third edition

We are delighted at the continued positive response we have received for *Psychiatry at a Glance* and at the many translations that have appeared in recent years. As before, this third edition is targeted primarily at medical students. We hope and intend that it helps them acquire the core psychiatric knowledge and skills specified within their new curricula and to foster positive attitudes to people with mental illness and their families. We have undertaken a comprehensive revision of all the existing chapters taking feedback both from young doctors and from specialists in the specific areas covered. We have also added several more questions. These are intended as a revision aid and we have therefore retained the format and thematic grouping which we acknowledge are no longer often used for examination purposes. We have also added a chapter on clinical examination technique.

The feedback we have received suggests that *Psychiatry at a Glance* is equally useful to nurses, social workers, psychologists, mental health workers and psychiatric trainees. We have tried to consider the needs of all these groups of readers in preparing the new edition.

As before, we owe a tremendous debt of gratitude to the many colleagues who have given constructive feedback. We therefore take this opportunity of thanking Profs Christodoulou, Gunn King, Kohen, Nutt, Salkovskis and Scott, Drs Abou-Saleh, Davies, Dein, Eapen, Groves, Hashmi, Hassiotis, Killaspy, Livingston, Norton, Orrell, Ring, Schmidt, Sensky, Shergill, Sturgeon, Thinn, Turner and Walker for giving up their time, and for their helpful comments. Responsibility for any errors and inaccuracies remains, of course, entirely ours.

We would like to thank Philippa Katona and John Ludgate for their patience and support on which we continue to rely.

Cornelius Katona
Mary Robertson
December 2004

Introduction to the first edition

We have written *Psychiatry at a Glance* at the instigation of many of our students, with the intention of providing a text that is concise, easily portable and enjoyable to read. The book summarizes the content of a comprehensive lecture course in psychiatry. It is targeted primarily at clinical undergraduate medical students doing their psychiatry attachment and revising for final MB examinations. It should also be useful for psychiatric trainees revising for their MRCPsych Part 1 (or equivalent first specialist examination).

We have both been MB final (and MRCPsych Part 1) examiners for several years, as well as being involved in the design and delivery of the UCL Medical School undergraduate and postgraduate psychiatry courses. We are confident of having provided all the information content relevant to the psychiatry element of the GMC 'core' undergraduate medical curriculum. The diagrams encapsulate all a medical student needs to know in order to pass—and should also help in last minute revision! The text supplements this sufficiently to provide enough for a student to do well.

We are also aware that, as psychiatric care moves into the community, a basic knowledge of psychiatry is increasingly important for a variety of clinical practitioners. *Psychiatry at a Glance* should provide a useful introduction to the specialty for psychiatric nurses (especially doing Project 2000 and postgraduate courses), for psychologists and social workers (in training and in clinical practice), and for general practitioners finding themselves in the psychiatric front line.

We have been encouraged throughout the writing of the book by students and colleagues (at UCL Medical School and elsewhere) alike. We owe a particular debt of gratitude to those who have taken the time to criticize individual chapters: Profs Barnes and Dinan; Drs Alcorn, Allen, Appleby, Barnes, Bhugra, Chesser, Collis, Cookson, Dein, Eapen, Feinmann, Freeman, Gardner, Jackson, Kahle, Kennedy, Livingston, McCarthy, Norton, Read, Ring, Orrell, Stansfeld, Sturgeon and Tannock; Jamie Arkel, Gina Hossain, Cheryl Moore, Paul de Keyser and Pippa Vincent. The content has been much improved by their criticism, although responsibility for any errors remains, of course, our own. We hope that you, the reader, will also feel able to offer suggestions for improvements to future editions. We would also like to thank John Ludgate for his support and encouragement.

Finally, we owe an enormous debt of gratitude to Philippa Katona, the GP on the Clapham omnibus, who has offered inestimable tolerance and support during the many evenings of writing, and helped ensure that both text and diagrams were much more relevant and comprehensible than they would otherwise have been.

Cornelius Katona
Mary Robertson
London

1 The psychiatric history and mental state examination (MSE)

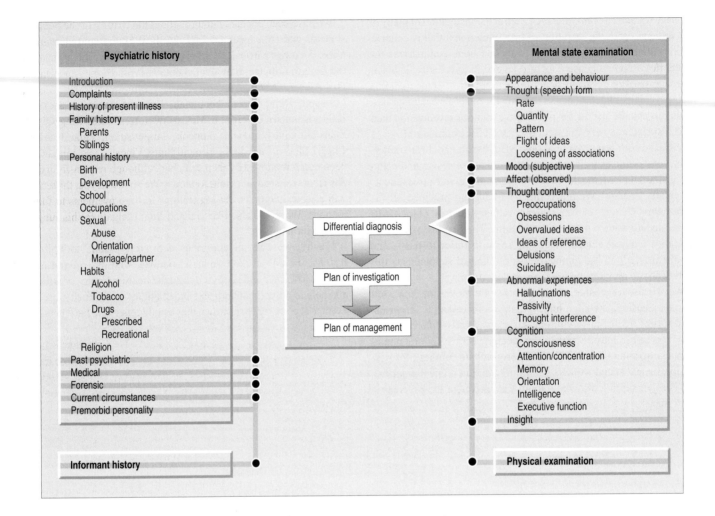

In taking a psychiatric history and assessing the mental state, it is crucial both to establish and maintain rapport and to be systematic in obtaining the necessary information. The outline below is intended as a schema for written documentation. Greater flexibility is clearly required during the interview.

The psychiatric history

The history begins with an *introduction* noting the patient's name, age, marital status, occupation, ethnic origin, religion and circumstances of referral. Then follows the *complaint* (in the patient's own words) and the *history of the present illness* (duration, precipitating factors, effect on interpersonal relationships, working capacity and details of treatment to date). In the *family history*, note parents'/siblings' ages, occupations, physical and mental health and relationships with the patient. If a relative is deceased, note the cause of death and the patient's age at the time of death. Enquiry is made into family history of psychiatric illness ('nervous breakdowns'), suicide, drug/alcohol abuse and forensic encounters.

The *personal history* begins with the patient's *early life and development* including details of the pregnancy (? planned) and birth (especially complications). Any serious illnesses, separations

in childhood or delays in development are noted. The childhood home environment is described (geographical situation, atmosphere) as are details of school (academic achievements, relationships with peers, teachers). The occupational history should list jobs, reasons for change, work satisfaction, relationships with colleagues. Document details of sexual practices (past/present abuse, sexual orientation, difficulties, satisfaction), relationships, marriage (duration, details of partner, children) and, in the case of women, menstrual pattern, contraception, miscarriages, stillbirths and terminations of pregnancy.

Previous psychiatric history (dates of illnesses, symptoms, diagnoses, treatments, hospitalizations) and *past medical and surgical history* are obtained. The patient's alcohol, drug (prescribed and recreational) and tobacco *consumption* and any *forensic* history are recorded. The patient's attitude to and practice of religion, politics and hobbies are noted. The *premorbid personality* (e.g. character, social relations) and finally, details of the present circumstances (accommodation, occupation, financial details), are described.

The MSE

The patient's *appearance and behaviour* are documented, including general health, demeanour, manner, rapport, eye contact, degree of cooperation, cleanliness, clothing, self-care, facial expression, posture, motor activity, which may be excessive (agitation) or decreased (retardation), abnormal movements (tics, chorea, tremor), stereotypy (purposeless), mannerisms (goal-directed, understandable), gait abnormality or striking physical features.

Speech is described in terms of rate, quantity (increased = pressure [often with associated 'flight of ideas']; decreased = poverty), and pattern (spontaneity, coherence, rationality, directness [to the point or discursive] and perseveration [repeating words or topics]). Abnormal words (neologisms), puns or rhymes should be noted, giving verbatim examples if abnormal. Abnormal *form of thought* may be deduced, for example where connections between statements are difficult to follow ('loosening of associations'). The patient's subjective experience of thought may be abnormal as in thought block (thoughts disappear: 'my mind goes blank').

Changes in *mood and affect* are the commonest symptoms of psychiatric disorder, but also occur in physical illness and in healthy people at times of adversity. *Mood* refers to subjective emotion as experienced by the individual, while *affect* is the observed (and often more transient) external manifestation of that emotion. Mood has been compared to climate, and affect to weather. Abnormalities of affect include blunting, lability, perplexity and suspiciousness. Abnormal mood states include depression, elation, euphoria (unconcerned contentment), anxiety and anger. It should be noted whether mood is consistent with thoughts and actions, or 'incongruous'.

Disorders of *thought content* include non-psychotic phenomena such as obsessional ideas (recurrent thoughts, feelings, images or impulses which are intrusive, persistent, senseless, unwelcome but recognized as the patient's own [in contrast to delusions]) and phobias (fear/anxiety which is out of proportion to the situation, cannot be reasoned or explained away and leads to avoidance behaviour). Suicidal ideation (thoughts) and intent (plans) are crucial.

Abnormal beliefs include overvalued ideas (abnormal beliefs or intense preoccupations, firmly held but comprehensible in the light of the subject's past experience and culturally shared belief systems). An example of this would be an intense but non-delusional feeling of guilty responsibility following bereavement. Ideas of reference are when the patient feels that other people look at or talk about him/her because they notice things about him/her, but insight (see below) is retained. Delusions (fixed, false, firmly held beliefs out of keeping with the patient's culture, unaltered by evidence to the contrary, and for which the patient has no insight) may be primary (no discernible connection with any previous experience or mood; autochthonous) or secondary (e.g. to mood). Passivity feelings are when the patient experiences outside control of or interference with his/her actions, feelings, perceptions and thoughts (thought interference). The latter may involve thought insertion or withdrawal (thoughts being put into and taken out of the person's mind) and thought broadcast (the experience that others can hear or read the individual's mind/thoughts).

Abnormal experiences include depersonalization—the unpleasant experience of subjective change, feeling detached, unreal, empty within, unable to feel emotion, watching oneself from outside (e.g. 'it feels as if I am cut off by a pane of glass'). The related phenomenon of derealization is the experience of the world or people in it seeming lifeless ('as if made out of cardboard').

Abnormalities of perception include illusions (distortions of perception of an external stimulus, e.g. interpreting a curtain cord as a snake); hallucinations (perceptions in the absence of an external stimulus which are experienced both as true and coming from the outside world); and pseudo-hallucinations (internal perceptions with preserved insight). Hallucinations can occur in any sensory modality, although auditory and visual are commonest. Some auditory hallucinations occur in normal individuals, when falling asleep (hypnagogic) or on waking (hypnopompic).

Within the *cognitive assessment*, the following are noted: level of consciousness, memory (long- and short-term, immediate recall), orientation in time (day, date, time), place, person, attention and concentration, general knowledge and intelligence. Educational background must be taken into account.

An assessment of the patient's *insight* (degree of correct understanding a patient has of his/her condition and its cause as well as his/her willingness to accept treatment) is made, after which the examiner notes his/her *reaction to the patient*.

The *physical examination* should focus on identifying (or excluding) conditions of which a suspicion has been raised in the history and MSE and/or with a known association with psychiatric illness.

In presenting a case, the history and MSE should be followed by a justified statement of diagnosis (or differential diagnosis), and concluded by a summary of possible aetiological factors (predisposing, precipitating and maintaining) and a plan for further investigation and management.

2 Diagnosis and classification in psychiatry

DSM–IV-TR (multiaxial)	ICD–10 (categorical)	Dimensional
Axis I	F90–98 Onset specific to childhood and adolescence	
Diagnoses before adulthood	F00–09 Organic	
Organic		
Secondary to medical condition		
Substance-related	F10–19 Due to psychoactive substance use	Psychotic
Schizophrenia, etc.	F20–29 Schizophrenia, etc.	
Mood	F30–39 Mood (affective)	
Anxiety		
Somatoform	F40–48 Neurotic, stress-related and somatoform	
Factitious		
Dissociative		
Eating	F50–59 Associated with physiological disturbances	
Sleep		
Impulse-control		
Adjustment		Neurotic
Axis II		
Personality disorders	F60–69 Personality and behaviour	Psychoticism
		Intraversion/extraversion
		Neuroticism
Mental retardation	F70–79 Mental retardation	
	F80–89 Psychological development	
Axis III		
General medical conditions		
Axis IV		
Psychosocial and environmental problems		
Axis V		
Global assessment of functioning		

History

Diagnoses and classifications in psychiatry have undergone tremendous changes in the last 40 years. Before the 1950s, diagnoses were not only unreliable, but even had meanings that varied considerably across the world. By the end of that decade, 'antipsychiatrists' including Laing and Szasz had started to suggest that diagnoses and classification in psychiatry should be abandoned, together with the concept of mental illness. In the 1960s, the World Health Organization (WHO) instigated a world-wide programme (>30 countries) aimed at improving diagnosis and classification of mental disorders, fostering research into the reliability of diagnosis and classification. The mental health section of the International Classification of Diseases (ICD) is currently in its 10th edition (ICD-10). The American Psychiatric Association developed its own classificatory system, the Diagnostic and Statistical Manual of Mental Disorders (DSM); the current classification, DSM-IV-TR, was published in 2000.

The concept of mental illness

The idea that illnesses of the mind were fundamentally different to other illnesses dates from the end of the eighteenth century, when Cartesian dualism was the dominant philosophy. In fact this is an artificial separation as physical illnesses affect the mind and vice versa. Pain is a purely psychological phenomenon, and fear and other emotions are important in the genesis of hypertension, asthma and other illnesses. This separation is apparent in the commonly held health belief that people with mental illness are in some way to blame for their illness, while people with physical illness are not, and in the increased stigma surrounding mental illness.

In general medicine, a distinction is made between 'disease' (objective physical pathology and known aetiology) and 'illness' (subjective distress). For most psychiatric conditions, aetiology is 'multifactorial', and there is no demonstrable pathology. Therefore, the term 'disorder' is often preferred to describe 'a clinically recognisable set of symptoms and behaviour' (ICD-10). The advent of new techniques (e.g. neuroimaging) may, however, result in the emergence of definable psychiatric diseases.

Aims and purposes

The purpose of classification is to identify groups of patients who are similar in their clinical features, course of disease, outcome and response to treatment. This not only aids individual clinical management but also provides patterns of treatment response and prognosis which can be extrapolated to future patients. Disease classification also facilitates communication with medical, legal and other professionals, and research into the aetiology, prevention and treatment of psychiatric conditions. For many psychiatric symptoms, there is a continuum, for example from normal sadness to severe depression. It is necessary to define a level of subjective distress greater in severity and/or duration than occurs in normal human experience, or above which treatment is beneficial.

Psychiatry is more concerned than other branches of medicine with classification, because there are generally no physical signs, diagnostic tests or specific aetiologies to confirm diagnoses. Therefore the accuracy of diagnoses is solely dependent on how they are defined. Two measures of diagnostic accuracy commonly examined are the *reliability* (reproducibility between different settings) and *validity* (extent to which people who have the disorder are identified by the diagnostic criteria). Validity is more difficult to confirm but attempts have been made, including the examination of consistency of symptom patterns and demonstration of consistent treatment responses, long-term prognoses, genetic and biological correlates. *Discriminating symptoms* occur commonly in a defined syndrome, but rarely in other syndromes (e.g. thought broadcast/schizophrenia [see Chapter 3]), while *characteristic symptoms* occur frequently in the defined syndrome but also occur in other syndromes (e.g. depressed mood, which though common in depressive illness also occurs in schizophrenia, alcoholism, etc.). *Operational definitions* mean the specification of precise inclusion and exclusion criteria.

Types of classification

Traditionally, mental disorder is differentiated into *mental retardation* (learning disability, in which features of the disorder have been present from birth or an early age), *personality disorder* (usually present from childhood or adolescence onwards), *mental illness* (where there is an identifiable onset of illness preceded by normal functioning), *adjustment disorder* (less severe than mental illness, occurring in relation to stressful events or changed circumstances), *disorders of childhood* and *other disorders* (those which do not fit into any other group, including behavioural disorders and substance misuse). Mental illness has in turn traditionally been differentiated into *organic* and *functional (psychotic and neurotic)* types.

Three main ways of classifying include the *categorical, dimensional* and *multiaxial* types. *Categorical systems* describe a group of entirely separate conditions, which are usually classified *hierarchically* so that each patient can receive one main diagnosis (organic psychoses take precedence over functional psychoses which take precedence over neuroses). The terms *psychosis* (with hallucinations and delusions, lacking insight [see Chapter 1] and a more severe form of illness) and *neurosis* (mental distress in the absence of hallucinations or delusions, insight retained and less

severe illness) are widely used and may be regarded as a categorical system. Within this system most depressive and anxiety disorders would fall within the neurotic category. *Dimensional systems* use a *continuum* rather than categories and have been used mainly to classify personality. For example, Eysenck has proposed three dimensions of personality: introversion/extraversion, neuroticism and psychoticism. A psychotic/neurotic continuum for major mental illness has been suggested by Kendell. Finally, *multiaxial systems* categorize the patient on *several axes*, rating patients on several separate categorical systems each measuring a different aspect (e.g. psychiatric diagnosis, personality, intelligence).

Systems of classification

The two main current systems of classification include the *ICD* and the *DSM*. ICD-10 is a *uniaxial system* which attempts to standardize using *descriptive definitions* of the syndromes and operational criteria, as well as producing directives on differential diagnosis. DSM-IV-TR, a *multiaxial* system, relies on operational criteria (rather than descriptive definitions). It states which symptoms need to be present (often quantifying their number and requiring a specific length of time for symptoms to be present) as well as exclusion criteria. DSM-IV-TR includes the following: axis I = clinical syndromes and other conditions that may be a focus of clinical attention; axis II = personality disorders and mental retardation (the latter classified by severity rather than aetiology); axis III = general medical conditions; axis IV = psychosocial and environmental problems; axis V = global assessment of functioning. ICD-10, in contrast, is more reliant on clinical description, although a research supplement has been produced which provides operational criteria more similar to those of DSM-IV-TR.

ICD-10 and DSM-IV-TR use broadly matching, although not always identical, major diagnostic categories as follows.

1 Disorders usually first diagnosed in infancy, childhood or adolescence (which may reflect developmental disorders, discrete illnesses or a combination of the two).

2 Delirium, dementia, amnestic and other cognitive disorders.

3 Mental disorders due to a general medical condition not elsewhere classified.

4 Psychoactive substance-related disorders.

5 Schizophrenia (including schizotypal, delusional and other psychotic disorders).

6 Mood (affective) disorders.

7 Anxiety (neurotic) disorders.

8 Somatoform, factitious and dissociative disorders.

9 Sexual and identity disorders.

10 Eating disorders.

11 Sleep disorders.

12 Impulse-control disorders.

13 Adjustment disorders.

3 Schizophrenia: phenomenology and aetiology

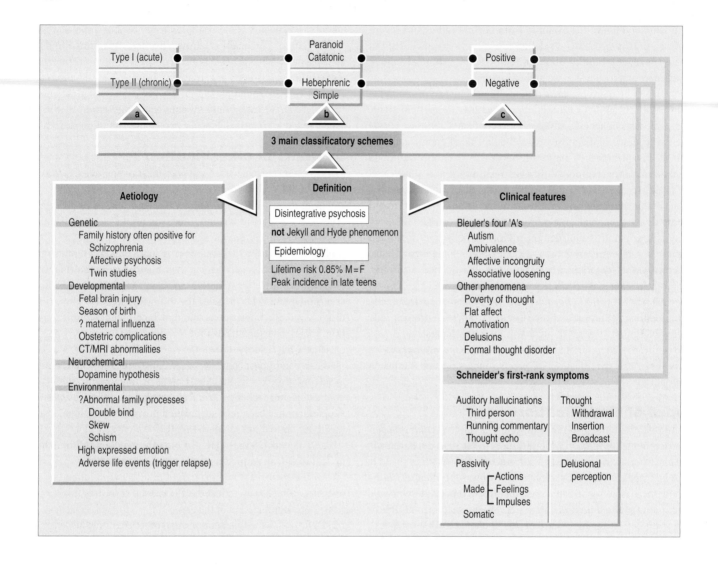

Introduction, history and definition

Many lay people misconceive schizophrenia as a 'split personality' or 'Jekyll and Hyde' phenomenon in which the individual can behave quite normally at times but is liable to change suddenly and become bizarre or dangerous. In fact, schizophrenia (literally 'split mind') is a disintegrative psychosis, characterized by the 'splitting' of normal links between perception, mood, thinking, behaviour and contact with reality. This results in delusions (fixed, false, beliefs not in keeping with their culture); hallucinations (perceptions without stimuli, e.g. hearing voices); disorganized thinking/speech (e.g. incoherence) and behaviour; negative symptoms (e.g. affective flattening); and social and/or occupational dysfunction. Emil Kraepelin (1893) suggested the distinction between bipolar affective disorder (manic–depressive illness), where normal function was regained between periods of relapse, and the term 'dementia praecox', characterized by the irreversible deterioration of mental functions (e.g. withdrawal, self-neglect and bizarre behaviour). This corresponds broadly to current concepts of schizophrenia.

Classification

The DSM-IV-TR classification suggests four main types: *paranoid* (delusions, auditory hallucinations); *catatonic* (motor immobility [e.g. stupor], excessive activity [excitement], rigidity, posturing [e.g. waxy flexibility = maintaining strange postures], echolalia [copying speech], echopraxia [copying behaviours]); *disorganized* (*hebephrenic*) (early onset, thought incoherence, disorganized behaviour, blunted or incongruous affect); and *undifferentiated* (*simple*) (deterioration, defect state). Other classification systems have proposed subtypes incorporating biological features and prognosis; Crow suggested *type I* (*acute* onset, positive symptoms [hallucinations, delusions], normal brain ventricular size, good prognosis, good response to neuroleptics, dopamine abnormalities) and *type II* (*chronic*, negative symptoms [e.g. flat affect], enlarged ventricles, poor prognosis, poor response to neuroleptics, neurone loss). Symptoms can be divided into three main factors: *positive* (hallucinations, delusions); *negative* (poverty of speech, flat affect, avolition [poor motivation]); and *cognitive* (poor attention and memory). There are overlaps between different typologies and, in any case, few patients fit neatly into one type only or only suffer from one symptom cluster.

Epidemiology

Schizophrenia occurs in 15–20/100 000 individuals per year, with a lifetime morbidity risk of 0.85% (male = female) and a peak incidence in late teens or early adulthood.

Clinical features

Classic symptoms include *Bleuler's four 'A's*: **A**utism (withdrawal from reality into an inner fantasy world); **A**mbivalence (coexistence of conflicting ideas, feelings); **A**ffective incongruity (affect and thoughts disassociated, e.g. smiling when discussing something sad, or blunting [flat]); and **A**ssociative loosening ('thought disorder', i.e. loosening of logical connections between thoughts).

Schneider's first-rank symptoms (SFRS) include specific types of auditory hallucination (third person discussing the patient, making a running commentary on the patient); thought echo (hearing one's own thoughts out loud [*echo de la pensée*]); thought withdrawal (thoughts taken out of head); thought insertion (thoughts put into mind); thought broadcast (thoughts available to others; the patient thinking everyone is thinking in unison with him/her); passivity (made acts, feelings, impulses, i.e. being controlled by outside forces); somatic passivity (bodily sensations controlled from without, e.g. blood boils after being struck by lightning); and delusional (apophanous) perception (attribution of a new meaning [with delusional intensity], usually self-referential, to a normally perceived object and often preceded by delusional mood [altered affect of fear, e.g. 'I heard a police siren and knew I had been appointed one of God's prophets', perplexity, foreboding, ecstasy, 'something going on around me']). Schneider considered SFRS diagnostic of acute schizophrenia if organic conditions were excluded. In fact, 8% of patients with non-schizophrenic functional psychoses have one or more SFRS, and 20% of people with chronic schizophrenia never show them. Second-rank symptoms, which are less diagnostically specific, include catatonic behaviour, secondary delusions and other hallucinations.

Other characteristic features of schizophrenia include poverty of thought (decreased thoughts and speech), flat (blunted) or incongruous affect, amotivation and delusions (often bizarre).

Formal thought disorder (e.g. loosening of associations, i.e. getting off the bus is successful because coffee is best), 'Knight's move thinking' (wandering off the point), neologisms (new words, or ordinary words used in a special way), concrete thinking (inability to deal with abstract ideas) and word salad (jumbled nonsense) are all found in schizophrenia.

Delusions may be primary (arising *de novo*, e.g. 'I am God') or secondary (arising from another morbid experience, e.g. hallucinations, passivity or mood). The content of delusions is dependent on social and cultural backgrounds (e.g. a religious person believing him/herself God, a doctor believing X-rays are being beamed into his/her house by the neighbours). Delusions in schizophrenia are usually systematized and often bizarre. Content is frequently persecutory (some individual or group is out to harm them, e.g. by poisoning), or of reference (e.g. patient is mentioned on TV news or knows that people are talking about him/her). It is important to be clear about the distinction between the term 'paranoid' (which refers to self-referential, i.e persecutory or grandiose, beliefs) and persecutory. Delusions may be of marital infidelity (incorrect beliefs of partner being unfaithful), grandiosity (patients believing they are God, Monarch, Napoleon), or nihilism (belief that their brain does not exist).

Both DSM-IV-TR and ICD-10 have *operational criteria* for schizophrenia which specify the presence of specific symptoms for certain lengths of time, and exclude other major disorders (e.g. depression).

Aetiology

There is a strong suggestion of *genetic factors* as aetiologically significant in schizophrenia, with a positive *family history* of schizophrenia and affective psychoses being reported with increased frequency in relatives of schizophrenics. *Twin studies* indicate that concordance rates are higher in monozygotic than dizygotic twins (MZ/DZ = 42 : 9%). *Adoptive studies* show that adopted-away offspring of schizophrenics have an increased (about 12%) chance of developing schizophrenia. No single gene has yet been identified. *Developmental* problems have also been invoked as aetiological, with fetal 'brain injury' (seasonality of birth [more births in winter]), low birth weight, order in large families, possibly maternal influenza during pregnancy, increased obstetric complications and perinatal injuries being suggested; brain computerized tomographic (CT) and magnetic resonance imaging (MRI) scans show increased ventricular size and small amounts of grey matter loss. 'Soft' neurological signs (e.g. abnormal movements, mixed-handedness) and temporal lobe epilepsy are associated with schizophrenia. The *dopamine hypothesis* of schizophrenia suggests dopamine excess or overactivity in mesolimbic pathways (amphetamines release dopamine and lead to psychosis; antipsychotics, which block dopamine receptors, treat psychosis successfully); increased dopamine receptors have been found at post-mortem. *Drug abuse*, particularly of stimulant drugs (amphetamines, cocaine) and cannabis has been shown to be linked with subsequent onset of schizophrenia in vulnerable individuals. *Abnormal family processes* have been suggested but not shown to be aetiologically significant. These include double-bind (parents convey two or more conflicting, incompatible messages at same time), skew (overprotective, intrusive, dominant mother; oversubmissive father), schism (hostility between parents), high expressed emotion (EE, relatives overinvolved or making excessive critical comments). People with schizophrenia experience an excess of *life events* in the 3 weeks before the onset of acute symptoms.

4 Schizophrenia: management and prognosis

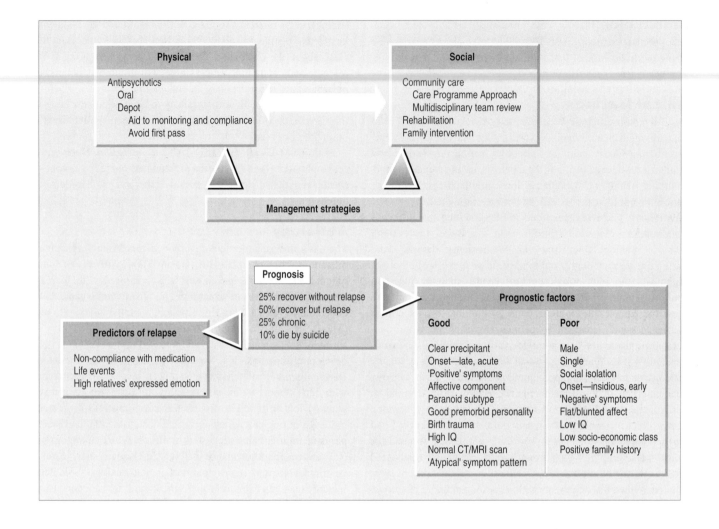

Management

Management includes ***antipsychotic*** (***neuroleptic***) medications (see Chapter 33) and ***psychosocial interventions***. Ideally, if the patient is in a first episode and/or requiring supervision, treatment should be supervised by a psychiatrist either informally (if the patient agrees), or under a 'Section' of the Mental Health Act if necessary (see Chapter 28). Admission to an in-patient unit may be necessary to alleviate the consequences of disordered behaviour and reduce the effects of psychosocial precipitants, for example family conflict, but also allows treatment (e.g. medication) to be initiated under supervision. In addition, patients with schizophrenia often lack family support and thus require admission, which may itself be therapeutic.

Antipsychotics are the drugs of choice. There is good evidence that they not only tranquillize and sedate the patient (non-specifically), but also have a specific therapeutic effect on the 'positive symptoms' in the acute episode (e.g. hallucinations, delusions, passivity phenomena, thought alienation). 'Atypical' antipsychotics are the preferred choice as they generally cause less side-effects,

and may improve negative symptoms and have an effect on low mood. If the patient is agitated, overactive or violent, he/she may require sedation (e.g. with typical antipsychotics or benzodiazepines). 'Typical' antipsychotics are also effective in treating mainly 'positive' symptoms. Medication may be administered ***orally***, ***intramuscularly*** or by long-acting ***depot injections*** (e.g. flupenthixol [Depixol]; fluphenazine [Modecate]; and the atypical medication risperidone [Risperdal]), which provide long-term prophylaxis, increase compliance, allow regular contact with either community psychiatric nurses (CPNs) or clinics and avoid first pass metabolism. Only clozapine, the prototypical atypical antipsychotic drug, has been shown to be effective in the treatment of refractory illness.

If the patient experiences extrapyramidal side-effects (e.g. dystonia, oculogyric crisis), anticholinergic drugs (e.g. procyclidine, benztropine) should be given immediately to reduce the extrapyramidal side-effects, making the patient more comfortable and rendering the antipsychotics more 'acceptable'. Regular antiparkinsonian drugs should be avoided as they cause unwanted side-effects (e.g. blurred vision, dry mouth), may be abused, and may worsen or provoke tardive dyskinesia (TD). TD may respond to the reduction/cessation of antipsychotics or to tetrabenazine but is irreversible in up to 50% of cases. Weight gain, cardiac arrythmias and diabetes may also be problematic during treatment with atypical antipsychotic drugs. People with schizophrenia can become depressed and may require antidepressant medication. Occasionally, *electroconvulsive therapy* (*ECT*) may be useful (e.g. catatonic stupor, excitement). After discharge from hospital, regular out-patient appointments are an important support as well as a facility for monitoring the patient's mental state and medication.

Psychotherapy (supportive) and counselling are important for all patients with schizophrenia and for their families and/or carers. Cognitive–behavioural techniques may be useful in helping patients cope with persistent delusions and hallucinations, and in rewarding appropriate behaviour patterns. Operant techniques may be helpful in patients with socially embarrassing or withdrawn behaviour. Family therapy helps the family reduce their excessive 'expressed emotion' (EE) and deal with separation from the patient and avoid relapse of the illness. Psychoanalysis is rarely useful.

Rehabilitation is an important part of treatment, and usually includes occupational therapy, counselling and supportive psychotherapy while in hospital. Social workers may also help with sorting out accommodation, finances, etc. (troubles which may adversely affect the patient's mental state). Institutionalization (with the handicaps it brings) must be avoided; therefore the patient should be encouraged to go on leave from hospital, have retraining in skills and employment and be discharged as soon as is practical. After discharge, further rehabilitation can take place at day hospitals, half-way houses, sheltered workshops and/or day centres. These are important for ensuring medication, providing recreation, activities and appropriate work experience. Both under and over-stimulation must be avoided.

It is important to note that a combination of antipsychotic medication, supportive psychotherapy and social measures is more efficacious than medication alone.

Community care is becoming increasingly important with the closing down of the large psychiatric hospitals in many parts of the world. Appropriate accommodation is important, and there may be a fine balance between independence and potential isolation; hostels or half-way houses are a good compromise. A concern about community care is that, in many parts of the world, it is being implemented without adequate financial and personnel resources; the more disadvantaged patients may well, in these instances, become vagrants or be imprisoned. Recent tragedies in the UK and other parts of the world have attracted media and government attention and resulted in new measures and legislations to deal with the problems of 'at risk' (e.g. of violence or suicide) in the community. The Care Programme Approach (CPA) in the UK emphasizes multidisciplinary team (MDT) work and regular patient review. Under the CPA, each patient is assigned a designated 'key worker' who may be any member of the MDT, such as the CPN or community psychiatric occupational therapist. This 'key worker' will visit the discharged patient, providing support, monitoring the mental state and treatment compliance, and helping with practical aspects of daily life (e.g. sorting out finances). Individuals at serious risk of suicide, self-neglect or serious violence may be placed on a supervision register and followed up very closely by 'key workers' who may instigate admission if the individual deteriorates sufficiently to cause concern.

Prognosis

One-quarter of patients with schizophrenia recover without a subsequent relapse, 50% recover but relapse in the future (often with increasingly severe residual symptoms) and 25% fail to recover at all, developing a chronic illness: 10% die by suicide. Suicide risk is higher in young men with persistent hallucinations or delusions, especially just before/during the first 3 months after discharge. Better prognosis is encountered in the developing world, which may be due to the social structure, family support or less stigma.

Good prognostic factors include a clear precipitant prior to the onset of the schizophrenic episode, older age at onset, an acute onset, 'positive' symptoms, a strong affective component (e.g. depressed), paranoid subtype, good premorbid personality, history of birth trauma, higher intelligence and a normal MRI/CT scan. Prognosis is also better with 'atypical' cases, for example schizoaffective disorder (illness typical of schizophrenia but with either a major depressive, manic or mixed episode, concurrent with symptoms of schizophrenia).

Poor prognostic factors include male gender, being single, social isolation, an insidious early onset without precipitants, negative symptomatology (e.g. amotivation), lack of affective component (flat, blunted affect), low IQ, low socio-economic class, abnormal premorbid personality and a positive family history of schizophrenia.

Factors that predict relapse include non-compliance with antipsychotic medication, adverse 'life events' (e.g. death of a close relative) and high EE (critical comments or overinvolvement in the family, measured during a standardized research interview), if contact is experienced for over 35 hours a week.

5 Depression

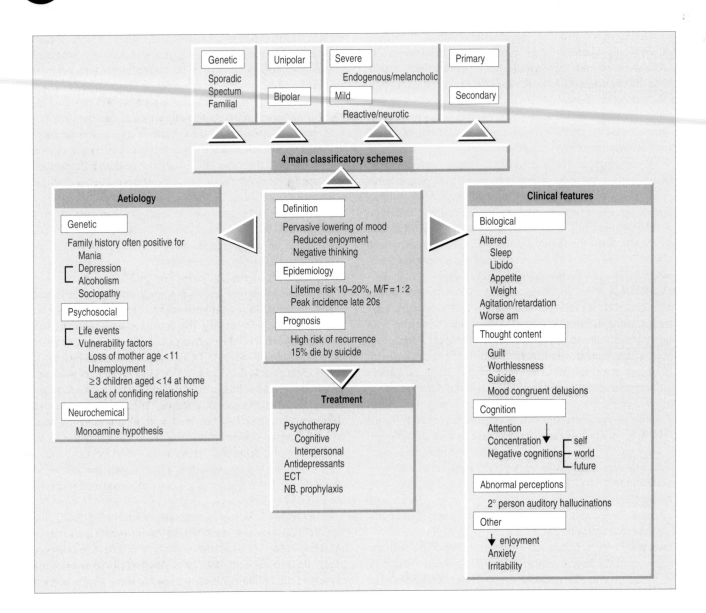

Definitions and classification

The most common feature of depression is a pervasive lowering of mood, although it is not essential for a diagnosis to be made (ICD-10). Most patients also experience loss of enjoyment (anhedonia) and negative patterns of thinking. There is, however, wide variation in symptomatology and in severity. This has resulted in considerable disagreement as to classification. Four main schemes have emerged. The best known of these proposes a dichotomy between 'endogenous' and 'neurotic' (also termed 'reactive') depression. The former is more severe, less likely to have external precipitants and is characterized by prominent 'biological' features (see below), whereas the latter is milder, more understandable in terms of external circumstances, more heterogeneous and may show symptomatic overlap with anxiety. In recent years the notion of a mild/severe continuum has largely replaced the 'endogenous'/'neurotic'

dichotomy. Depression may also be seen as bipolar (having a tendency to abnormal upswings as well as downswings of mood) versus unipolar (episodes of depression only); and secondary (associated with other psychiatric or physical illness) versus primary. The fourth classification is genetic, dividing depressions into 'familial' (positive family history of depression); 'spectrum' (positive family history of related conditions such as alcoholism and personality disorders) and 'sporadic' (no relevant family history).

The unipolar/bipolar and severe/mild distinctions are favoured in the current ICD-10 and DSM-IV-TR classifications (see Chapter 2).

Clinical features

Depressed mood, anhedonia and increased fatiguability are regarded as the most typical symptoms in the ICD-10 classification. Depression can be 'masked' by anxiety, excess consumption of alcohol, hypochondriacal preoccupations or irritability; such atypical presentations are particularly common in adolescence (ICD-10). The main biological changes involve sleep, appetite and libido. Sleep is reduced with a pattern of early waking and maximal lowering of mood in the morning (diurnal variation). Appetite is reduced with associated weight loss and, in severe cases, reluctance or refusal even to drink. Libido is reduced or absent. Anhedonia is accompanied by loss of motivation. Motor activity is often altered, with retardation (of speech and/or movement), agitation or both. In 'neurotic' depressions the pattern may be inverted with initial anxiety-related insomnia, subsequent oversleeping and increased appetite.

Thought content often includes negative, pessimistic thoughts about the self (i.e. low self-esteem), the world and the future (Beck's cognitive triad), thoughts of death or suicide and feelings of guilt and worthlessness. Cognitive function may be impaired, with reduced attention and/or concentration. Delusions and hallucinations are usually 'mood congruent'. The former will typically concern illness or death. The latter are relatively rare, usually auditory in the second person and accusing, condemning or urging suicide.

Differential diagnosis

Depression may be difficult to distinguish from normal sadness, particularly in the context of bereavement (see Chapter 8) or severe physical illness. The diagnosis depends on finding a pattern of characteristic features (as above) accompanying the low mood; and on the degree and duration of associated disability. Predominant anxiety symptoms may obscure the diagnosis of depression. Depressive retardation may be difficult to distinguish from the affective flattening of schizophrenia. Diagnosis of depression can be difficult in people abusing alcohol and illicit drugs, because withdrawal can mimic depression, but substance misuse can also be a symptom or aetiological factor in depressive illness.

Epidemiology

The lifetime risk of depression is about 10%, with rates almost doubled in women. First onset is typically in the third decade (earlier for bipolar disorder) with point prevalence higher in middle and old age. Depression is commoner in urban than in rural areas, and particularly in women from lower socio-economic classes.

Aetiology

A genetic contribution is evident in both twin and adoption studies, less markedly for unipolar than bipolar depression. Neurochemical and neuroendocrine mechanisms have been proposed. The dominant neurochemical theory is the 'monoamine hypothesis' based on the observations (in the 1960s) that monoamine (particularly noradrenaline and serotonin) metabolites in cerebrospinal fluid (CSF) and urine are reduced in depressed patients, and that antidepressants increase monoamine availability. This has been modified to emphasize changes in monoamine neuroreceptors (particularly β-adrenoreceptors and $5HT_2$ receptors) related to depression and to antidepressant treatment. The impact of increased monoamine availability on mood may be mediated by increased expression of neurotrophins, which are important in neuronal growth. Neuroen-

docrine abnormalities found in some depressed patients include hypercortisolaemia (and related impairment of dexamethasone-induced suppression of cortisol secretion), and impaired thyroid axis activity. Depression is also associated with characteristic sleep-electroencephalographic (EEG) changes and reduced frontal lobe blood flow.

The most important exogenous factors implicated are recent adverse life events (such as bereavement and deteriorating physical health), and parental loss and/or major stress or abuse in childhood (which appears to increase vulnerability to depression in response to life events). These factors may be involved in endogenous as well as neurotic depression. Adverse current social circumstances, especially unemployment and lack of a confiding relationship, may also increase such vulnerability. Several physical illnesses (most endocrine disorders, many cancers, some viral infections) are specifically associated with depression. Women appear particularly vulnerable to episodes of depression in the weeks following childbirth.

Management

Most depressive illnesses can be managed in the primary care setting, although many are undetected. Detection rates can be enhanced by remembering that depressed patients often present with other conditions, and/or by simple screening questionnaires. Management starts with risk assessment, in terms of self-neglect and, most importantly, suicide. Psychiatric referral is indicated if suicide risk is high, or if the depression is severe, unresponsive to initial treatment or recurrent. Comorbid physical illnesses or substance misuse problems should be addressed. Pharmacological treatments (see Chapter 33) include tricyclic and newer antidepressants (e.g. selective serotonin reuptake inhibitors [SSRIs]) and can have a 60–70% response rate, but frequently fail because of inadequate dosage, duration or compliance. Electroconvulsive therapy (ECT) is very effective in severe cases, particularly where delusions and/or retardation are present, and can be life saving if fluids and food are being refused. Refractory depression may respond to combination treatments such as lithium augmentation. Specific psychological techniques (including cognitive–behaviour therapy [CBT], interpersonal and problem-solving psychotherapy) have similar success rates to antidepressants in non-psychotic depression; CBT also has some prophylactic effect. Continuing antidepressants for at least 6 months after a first episode reduces relapse rate; in recurrent depression prophylactic effects have been demonstrated for up to 5 years.

Prognosis

Single episodes of depression usually last between 3 and 8 months; about 20% of patients remain depressed for 2 years or more. About 50% have recurrences; this rises to 80% in severe cases (such as in those requiring in-patient care). Recurrent episodes tend to become increasingly severe with shortening of disease-free periods, emphasizing the importance of prophylactic treatment. Lifetime suicide risk is 15% in severe depression but much lower in milder illness. Predictors of poor outcome include early onset, initial symptom severity and psychiatric or physical comorbidity.

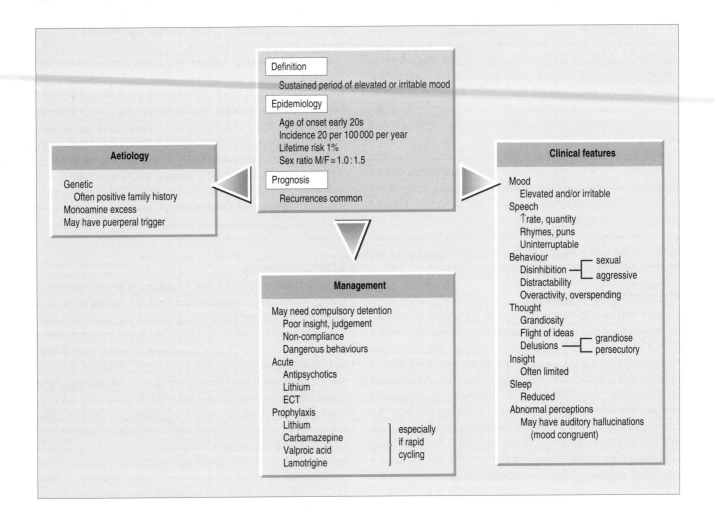

Definitions and classification

The bipolar affective disorders are characterized by recurrent episodes of altered mood and activity, involving upswings as well as downswings. Recent classificatory systems (DSM-IV-TR, ICD-10) have therefore had to define both individual episodes and patterns of recurrence. Individual episodes include major depressive episode (see Chapter 5); manic episode; hypomanic episode (less severe); and mixed episode, in which features of mania and major depression alternate rapidly. Patterns of recurrence can be classified as bipolar I disorder (with one or more manic or mixed episodes and, usually, one or more major depressive episodes); bipolar II disorder (recurrent major depressive and hypomanic but not manic episodes); and cyclothymic disorder, with chronic mood fluctuations over at least 2 years including individual episodes of hypomania (but not mania) and of depression insufficient in severity to meet major depression criteria.

Clinical features

The cardinal clinical feature of a manic episode is alteration in mood, which is often elated and expansive but may also be characterized by intense irritability. Associated features include increased psychomotor activity (rapid thinking and speech, distractibility, decreased need for sleep); decreased social inhibition and disregard for potentially painful consequences (sexual overactivity, over-spending, indulgence in poorly considered or inappropriate business, religious or political initiatives); and exaggerated optimism and inflated self-esteem, which may be reflected in grandiose delusions or hallucinations. Mood incongruent psychotic features may also be found; indeed, one or more Schneiderian first-rank symptoms (see Chapter 3) are occasionally present but may indicate a schizoaffective disorder. Heightened sensory awareness is common. More specific speech abnormalities include uninterruptibility and sound—rather than sense—triggered speech content (punning, clanging). Insight is often variable or absent. Manic and hypomanic episodes are distinguished on the basis that mania is more severe (causing marked work, social and/or interpersonal disruption) and usually necessitates hospitalization, whereas hypomania is less severe and disruptive and fewer clinical features are present.

Differential diagnosis

The most important differential diagnoses are organic. These include substance abuse (particularly amphetamines or cocaine) and mood abnormalities secondary to endocrine disturbance (idiopathic Cushing's syndrome or steroid-induced psychoses) or epilepsy. 'Secondary' mania or organic mood disorder may also be precipitated by severe physical illness (particularly stroke). Acute schizophrenia may present very much like mania: persecutory delusions are common in both, and the distinction between formal thought disorder and flight of ideas may be difficult. Other conditions to consider include attention-deficit hyperactivity disorder and transient psychoses induced by extreme stress. In both of these, elevation of mood is rare.

Epidemiology

The lifetime prevalence of bipolar disorder is about 1%, with a ratio of bipolar I/cyclothymia/bipolar II of about 2:2:1. The female/male ratio is about 1.5:1.0, the female excess being in the bipolar II group. Peak age of first onset is in the early 20s. Several studies have shown higher prevalence rates in higher social classes, probably reflecting differences in access to diagnosis and treatment.

Aetiology

There is clear evidence of a strong familial component. Rates of both bipolar disorder (including cyclothymia) and unipolar depression are commoner than expected in first-degree relatives of bipolar subjects. Both sex-linked and autosomal inheritance have been proposed. A number of neuroendocrine abnormalities have been described including hypercortisolaemia, increased aldosterone secretion and blunted growth hormone response to hypoglycaemia. The findings are less consistent than in depressive illness, and usually similar rather than opposite. Some studies suggest that manic episodes may be precipitated by severe stress. In particular, there is a markedly increased risk of manic episodes occurring in the early postpartum weeks; this may relate to dopamine receptor supersensitivity associated with precipitate postpartum falls in oestrogen and progesterone levels. Psychodynamic models of mania implicate denial of loss or loss-associated conflict in order to avoid depression, and/or loss of superego ('conscience') control.

Management

Acute mania almost invariably requires hospitalization. Since patients often lose insight early, this may require detention without consent, using appropriate mental health legislation. Exclusion of organic causes is vital. Antipsychotics (in similar dosage to that used in schizophrenia) form the mainstay of acute management of both mania and hypomania. Antipsychotics are effective both in controlling overactivity and agitation, and (somewhat more slowly) in reducing elation and disinhibition. Lorazepam may be useful for rapid tranquillization. Lithium is also effective as an acute antimanic agent, although it lacks the potential for very rapid behavioural control. In patients unresponsive to antipsychotics (particularly where extreme overactivity is a threat to physical health), electroconvulsive therapy (ECT) may be effective. Maintenance treatment with lithium has been shown in many controlled trials to reduce the frequency and severity of subsequent episodes. Its 'real-life' effectiveness is harder to demonstrate and probably depends on careful supervision and education enabling good compliance. Lithium therapy (which may also be useful in cyclothymia) requires comprehensive pre-initiation screening (including renal and thyroid function estimation) and regular monitoring in view both of its narrow therapeutic range and its long-term potential to induce hypothyroidism. A number of anticonvulsants (carbamazepine, valproic acid and lamotrigine) appear to be effective in preventing manic relapse, particularly where psychotic feelings have been prominent. Anticonvulsants may also be preferable to lithium where rapid cycling occurs (see below). Psychotherapeutic support is important in helping patients come to terms with their illness and their remorse at their past manic behaviour.

Prognosis

The lifetime prognosis following a single manic episode is poor, with 90% of patients having manic and/or depressive recurrences (averaging four episodes in 10 years). In bipolar I disorder, both frequency and severity of episodes tend to increase for the first four or five episodes, but tend subsequently to plateau. Long-term functional prognosis (work, family, etc.) is almost as poor as in schizophrenia. A minority develop 'rapid cycling', with four or more episodes a year; they have a particularly poor prognosis and seldom respond to lithium. There is an overall increase in premature mortality, only partially explained by a suicide rate of 10%. Successful lithium prophylaxis (reflecting self-selection for good prognosis as well as good response to lithium) not only modifies severity and duration of episodes, but appears to reduce both suicide and overall mortality. Prognosis for bipolar II disorder is better, although there remains a high suicide risk. Cyclothymia has a chronic course and an approximately 30% risk of developing full-blown bipolar disorder.

Suicide and deliberate self-harm (DSH)

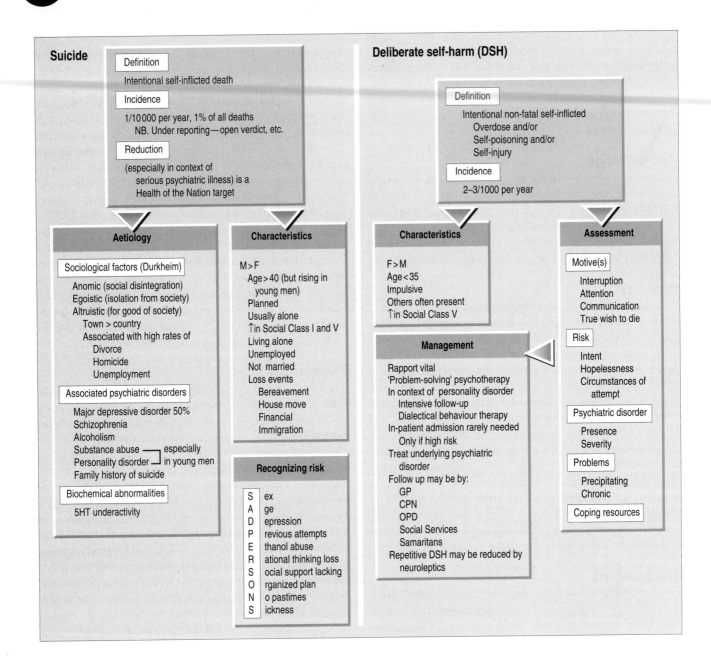

Suicide

Definition

Intentional self-inflicted death

Incidence

1/10 000 per year, 1% of all deaths
NB. Under reporting—open verdict, etc.

Reduction

(especially in context of
serious psychiatric illness) is a
Health of the Nation target

Aetiology

Sociological factors (Durkheim)

Anomic (social disintegration)
Egoistic (isolation from society)
Altruistic (for good of society)
  Town > country
  Associated with high rates of
  Divorce
  Homicide
  Unemployment

Associated psychiatric disorders

Major depressive disorder 50%
Schizophrenia
Alcoholism
Substance abuse —— especially
Personality disorder —┘ in young men
Family history of suicide

Biochemical abnormalities

5HT underactivity

Characteristics

M > F
Age > 40 (but rising in
  young men)
Planned
Usually alone
↑in Social Class I and V
Living alone
Unemployed
Not married
Loss events
  Bereavement
  House move
  Financial
  Immigration

Recognizing risk

S ex
A ge
D epression
P revious attempts
E thanol abuse
R ational thinking loss
S ocial support lacking
O rganized plan
N o pastimes
S ickness

Deliberate self-harm (DSH)

Definition

Intentional non-fatal self-inflicted
  Overdose and/or
  Self-poisoning and/or
  Self-injury

Incidence

2–3/1000 per year

Characteristics

F > M
Age < 35
Impulsive
Others often present
↑in Social Class V

Management

Rapport vital
'Problem-solving' psychotherapy
In context of personality disorder
  Intensive follow-up
  Dialectical behaviour therapy
In-patient admission rarely needed
  Only if high risk
Treat underlying psychiatric
  disorder
Follow up may be by:
  GP
  CPN
  OPD
  Social Services
  Samaritans
Repetitive DSH may be reduced by
  neuroleptics

Assessment

Motive(s)

Interruption
Attention
Communication
True wish to die

Risk

Intent
Hopelessness
Circumstances of
  attempt

Psychiatric disorder

Presence
Severity

Problems

Precipitating
Chronic

Coping resources

The assessment and acute management of DSH is probably the most critical psychiatric task facing the non-psychiatrist—particularly the (relatively inexperienced) medical house officer or casualty officer. Recognition of suicide risk is, together with better detection and management of psychiatric illness as a whole, crucial in reducing the suicide rate which, in the UK, has been identified as a National Health target.

Definitions

Suicide may be defined as intentional self-inflicted death; DSH represents intentionally self-inflicted harm without a fatal outcome.

Suicide
Epidemiology

International suicide rates vary widely, with the highest incidence in Hungary, the former Soviet Union and Finland. There are about 5000 suicides per year in England and Wales, an annual incidence of approximately 1/10 000 and representing about 1% of all deaths. Suicide rates in the UK are about three times higher in men than in women. Suicide rates in young men have recently risen sharply in most developed countries; highest rates are nonetheless found in older men.

Aetiology

Factors implicated in the aetiology of suicide can be classified as social, biological and psychiatric. Durkheim's social model described two main types of suicide: anomic and egoistic. *Anomic* suicide reflects a society's disintegration and loss of shared values; this is reflected in positive correlations between rates of suicide and of unemployment and homicide, reductions in suicide rate in wartime (social unity in adversity) and in Roman Catholic countries, and in the higher suicide rates in urban than rural communities. The relationship between suicide and unemployment is also found at the individual level, with job loss in men being associated with increased suicide risk both in themselves and their spouses. Some of this association is, however, explained by the increased risk of unemployment in the mentally ill. *Egoistic* suicide involves individuals' separation from otherwise cohesive social groups and finds some reflection in the higher suicide rates following bereavement and moving house, in immigrants, and in people living alone and divorced or single, compared to people who are married. A further social factor is availability of means: high rates in the USA have been linked to ease of obtaining firearms; UK rates fell sharply when toxic coal gas was replaced by (relatively) harmless natural gas. A positive family history of suicide is associated with increased suicide risk. A large proportion of completed suicides have consulted their general practitioners (GPs) in the weeks prior to suicide, highlighting the need to recognize people at risk and consequent prevention. Although no consistent biological correlate of suicide has been found, evidence both from brain and cerebrospinal fluid (CSF) studies in suicides and suicide attempters (particularly those using violent means) suggests that serotonergic underactivity (as reflected in levels of 5HT and its metabolites, as well as in 5HT receptors and uptake sites) may be involved.

Perhaps the strongest association with suicide is psychiatric illness, with rates increased 50-fold in psychiatric in-patients, and retrospective 'psychiatric autopsy' studies suggesting that a specific psychiatric diagnosis can be made in almost all suicides. Specific diagnoses implicated include major depression (with a lifetime suicide risk of 15%), schizophrenia (10%), alcoholism (3–4%), and (less consistently) personality disorder (present in 30–60% of completed suicides), anorexia nervosa, substance misuse and obsessive–compulsive disorder (OCD). The relationship between depression and suicide is strongest in old age. In contrast, the recent increase in suicide rates in young men is associated with personality disorders and substance abuse. Suicide rates are also increased in people with chronic painful illnesses.

The acronym 'SAD PERSONS' is an *aide-mémoire* for risk factors in suicides: **S**ex, **A**ge, **D**epression, **P**revious attempts, **E**thanol abuse, **R**ational thinking loss (particularly psychosis), **S**ocial support lacking, **O**rganized plan, **N**o pastimes and **S**ickness (with special attention to medical disorders that have been shown to increase risk).

DSH

Epidemiology and correlates

DSH is a much commoner event than completed suicide, with an annual incidence of 2–3/1000 in the UK, where (in contrast to the USA) most cases involve drug overdose rather than physical self-injury. Unlike completed suicide, DSH is commoner in women and the under 35s. DSH is commoner in lower social classes and in the single and divorced. Like suicide, DSH is associated with psychiatric illness, particularly depression (usually mild) and personality disorder.

Assessment

The immediate priority is medical stabilization. Subsequent psychiatric assessment involves establishing a rapport (essential if the DSH is to be a springboard to appropriate management) and necessitating a suspension of the assessor's pejorative judgments. Relevant interview topics include identification of motive(s), acute and chronic problems and associated coping strategies, and of current psychiatric illness. DSH is often precipitated by undesirable life events. In most cases, its motive can be understood in terms of one or more of a desire to *interrupt* a sequence of events seen as both inevitable and undesirable; a need for *attention* or to *communicate* (decoding and transmission of such communications may itself be effective in reducing subsequent risk); and a true *wish to die*. The latter, although probably the single best indicator of high subsequent risk of suicide, is seldom either unequivocal or stable. Subjects at high risk have a clinical profile more characteristic of suicide than of DSH; specific indicators of high risk include leaving a suicide note, continued determination to die, marked feelings of hopelessness, clear evidence of psychiatric illness (particularly severe depression) and an attempt carefully prepared with precautions against discovery and/or high lethality risk, either objectively or as imagined by the patient. In addition, risk is higher in older, male, unemployed or socially isolated subjects. Risk of repeated non-fatal DSH is highest in subjects of low social class, with antisocial personality disorder, no work and/or a criminal record and in substance abusers.

Options for management

The objectives of DSH management are to decrease short-term risk of repetition and of completed suicide, to initiate or continue treatment of any underlying psychiatric illness (NB. consider safety in overdose when prescribing antidepressants) and to address ongoing social difficulties. A good first step is to agree with the patient what their problems are, and what immediate interventions are both feasible and acceptable to them. Such a 'contract' can include a promise not to repeat any DSH. Only a small minority (usually where social support is lacking) need in-patient admission, although where suicide risk is high, compulsory admission may be indicated. Out-patient department (OPD) brief psychotherapy (e.g. 'problem solving') may be helpful, as may referral to social services and/or voluntary agencies such as the Samaritans. In patients with affective disorder, lithium has been shown to reduce risk of both DSH and completed suicide. The frequency of repetitive DSH in the context of personality disorder may be reduced by simple cognitive (problem-solving) techniques, intensive follow-up and depot antipsychotics. Dialectical behaviour therapy (see Chapter 32) has been shown to reduce repetitive self-harm in the context of personality disorder.

Outcome

About 20% of self-harmers repeat their act within 1 year. Risk of actual suicide within 1 year is 1–2%, a 100-fold increase compared with the general population.

8 Stress reactions (including bereavement)

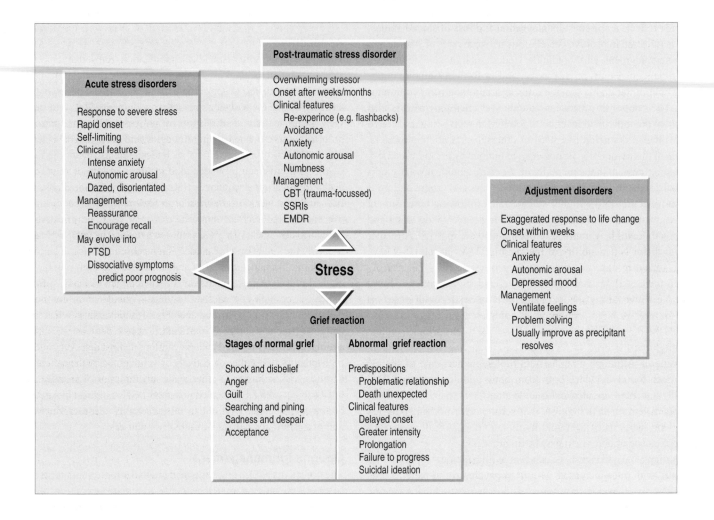

Acute stress disorders

Response to severe stress
Rapid onset
Self-limiting
Clinical features
    Intense anxiety
    Autonomic arousal
    Dazed, disorientated
Management
    Reassurance
    Encourage recall
May evolve into
    PTSD
    Dissociative symptoms
        predict poor prognosis

Post-traumatic stress disorder

Overwhelming stressor
Onset after weeks/months
Clinical features
    Re-experince (e.g. flashbacks)
    Avoidance
    Anxiety
    Autonomic arousal
    Numbness
Management
    CBT (trauma-focussed)
    SSRIs
    EMDR

Adjustment disorders

Exaggerated response to life change
Onset within weeks
Clinical features
    Anxiety
    Autonomic arousal
    Depressed mood
Management
    Ventilate feelings
    Problem solving
    Usually improve as precipitant
      resolves

Stress

Grief reaction

Stages of normal grief	Abnormal grief reaction
Shock and disbelief	Predispositions
Anger	Problematic relationship
Guilt	Death unexpected
Searching and pining	Clinical features
Sadness and despair	Delayed onset
Acceptance	Greater intensity
	Prolongation
	Failure to progress
	Suicidal ideation

Major psychological stress involves threat or loss. Reactions to a broad range of major stressors (physical or sexual assault, transport accidents, natural disasters, war) are often similar in nature and involve emotional responses (fear from threat and sadness at loss), physical symptoms (autonomic arousal and/or fatigue) and psychological responses which may be conscious (e.g. avoidance behaviour) or unconscious (e.g. denial or dissociation). Abnormal stress reactions represent exaggerated or maladaptive responses. They may be acute and self-limiting or more prolonged (post-traumatic stress disorder [PTSD], adjustment disorder or abnormal grief).

Acute stress disorders (ASDs)

ASDs are rapid onset, extreme responses (within minutes or hours) to sudden and severe stressful events. Intense subjective anxiety is accompanied by autonomic arousal (sweating, dry mouth, tachycardia, vomiting). Dissociative symptoms, which predict increased risk of PTSD, include feeling dazed and perplexed and wandering aimlessly. Purposeless overactivity, reduced sleep and nightmares are also common. Initial management involves helping to reorientate and 'ground' the individual. Practical support may be required in dealing with underlying difficulties (e.g. temporary rehousing after

a natural disaster). There is no evidence that anxiolytics or hypnotics are effective and they carry a risk of dependence. Sedating antidepressants are preferable. Increasing evidence suggests that brief cognitive–behaviour therapy (CBT) intervention improves outcome and reduces the rate of chronic PTSD. Persistence of symptoms for more than 1 month indicates the development of PTSD (see below). Enduring personality change, particularly loss of the ability to trust others, may occur after catastrophic stress.

Adjustment disorders (ADs)

ADs include a range of abnormal psychological responses to adversity. They may follow common life changes such as job loss, house move or divorce. The onset is usually within weeks of the stressful event and the duration is usually less than 6 months, unless there are factors leading to persistence (e.g. litigation). Symptoms are often similar to PTSD but may include a broad mixture of symptoms of anxiety (autonomic arousal, insomnia and irritability) and depression (sadness, tearfulness, worry). Biological features of depression are usually absent; indeed, the diagnosis should only be made where there are insufficient symptoms to justify a diagnosis of another specific anxiety or depressive disorder. Adjustment disorders usually improve following resolution of their precipitating cause.

Initial management may involve encouragement to ventilate feelings and to develop appropriate coping mechanisms. Such help may focus on 'problem solving' in which patients are encouraged to form strategies to deal with particular problems. Sometimes, formal CBT treatments are required.

Adjustment to chronic or terminal illness may manifest as anxiety, depression or exaggerated disability. There may be a sequence (similar to that in bereavement) of shock and denial (and search for an ever-elusive 'cure'), followed by anger, sadness and acceptance. Management involves adequate symptomatic (particularly pain) control, honest explanation, supportive psychotherapy and family counselling.

PTSD

The onset of PTSD may occur weeks, months or (rarely) years after the stressful experience (the nature of which may, as in ASD, include assault, accident, disaster or battle). DSM-IV-TR and ICD-10 require that the stressor be exceptionally severe for PTSD to be diagnosed. In DSM-IV-TR, the immediate element of shock is emphasized in the requirement for there to be an experience of intense fear, horror or helplessness. Duration of symptoms for 1 month is required to make the diagnosis. The characteristic features of PTSD involve:

1 *Persistent intrusive thinking or re-experiencing* of the trauma, such as traumatic memories, dissociative reliving experiences ('flashbacks') or nightmares.

2 *Avoidance* of reminders of the event (e.g. accident victims not going near the scene of the accident).

3 Persistent anxiety with autonomic symptoms, hypervigilance, sleep disturbance, irritability and poor concentration.

4 *Numbing* (loss of interest in everyday activities or loss of the ability to experience strong emotions such as love).

There is considerable symptomatic overlap between the avoidance and numbing symptoms of PTSD and depression (see Chapter 5); the latter may also be precipitated by extreme stress and may coexist with or be secondary to PTSD.

Risk for PTSD is proportional to the magnitude of the stressor, but may be greater following 'man-made' than natural disasters and if some stress continues. Lack of social support and the presence of other adversities at the time of the trauma are crucial vulnerability factors. Many PTSD victims recover over the first few months. If the syndrome persists over 1–2 years, then it may continue long-term, possibly for the rest of the victim's life—as in many Holocaust survivors. Trauma-focused CBT, eye movement desensitization and reprocessing (EMDR) and (second-line) antidepressant drugs (even in the absence of depressive disorder) have been shown to be effective. Debriefing (in which patients are encouraged to recall the stressful events in detail and supported through the associated emotions) immediately after the trauma was thought to prevent subsequent PTSD, but is not supported by the evidence. Alcohol or substance misuse may also be a long-term complication and should be considered.

Bereavement and grief

Bereavement is associated with increased mortality (from cardiovascular disease and cancer) and may precipitate depression and even suicide.

'Normal' grief often follows a recognizable sequence of stages that last for up to 2 years. The initial reaction to bereavement (lasting days or a few weeks) is of **shock and disbelief** with autonomic arousal but usually without psychological fear. There may be paroxysms of weeping. This may be followed by **anger** at being deserted by the deceased relative, and **guilt and self-blame** for not having done more for them. The next stage consists of **'searching' or 'pining'**, vivid dreams that the dead person is still alive and, often, pseudo-hallucinations (usually at night and always with preserved insight) of the dead person speaking to them. **Sadness and despair** follow this, accompanied by many features (poor sleep and appetite, social withdrawal) of depression. Finally, **acceptance** occurs that the deceased will not come back, accompanied by return of interests. Symptoms often recur briefly on anniversaries. The sequence of stages is often less clear-cut than this linear model suggests. Bereavement is also often characterized by jumbled feelings as people pass in and out of these stages of grieving.

'Abnormal' grief is characterized by delayed onset of grief, greater intensity of symptoms, or prolongation of the reaction. Suicidal ideas may be harboured during abnormal pining (a wish to be with the deceased) or despair. Abnormal grief is more likely where the relationship with the deceased was problematic (ambivalent or overinvolved), the death sudden, or normal grieving impeded by social constraints (e.g. 'having to put on a brave face for the children').

Normal grieving requires no specific management apart from support and encouragement to ventilate feelings and accept them as normal. Abnormal grief reactions may respond to CBT, encouraging structured review of the relationship and giving vent to the emotions produced. Antidepressants may be indicated if depressive symptoms are prominent and persistent. Significant suicidal ideation may warrant hospitalization.

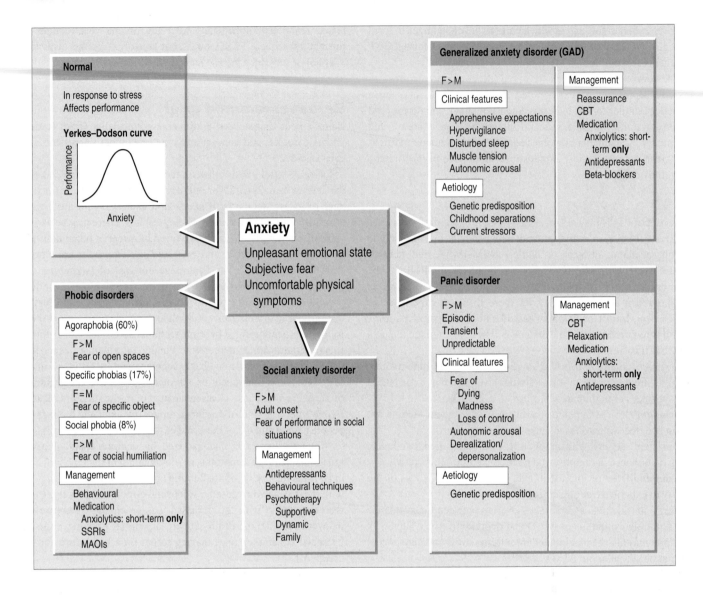

Definition and classification

Anxiety is an unpleasant emotional state accompanied by a subjective experience of fear, bodily discomfort and physical symptoms which may be accompanied by a feeling of impending threat or death in the future, and which may or may not be in response to a recognizable threat. The Yerkes–Dodson curve of anxiety against performance illustrates that anxiety can be beneficial up to a plateau of optimal function beyond which, with increasing anxiety, there is a marked deterioration in performance. Pathological anxiety can present in discrete attacks with no external stimulus (panic disorder), in discrete attacks with stimuli (phobias) or in a generalized, persistent state (generalized anxiety disorder [GAD]). Anxiety can, however, also occur as part of other disorders (e.g. depression).

Panic disorder

Panic disorder is characterized by recurrent episodic severe panic (anxiety) attacks (PAs) which occur unpredictably and are not restricted to any particular situation or set of circumstances (although certain situations such as being in crowds may become associated with them). PAs are discrete periods of intense fear, impending doom or discomfort, accompanied by characteristic symptoms, palpitations, tachycardia, a pounding heart, sweating, trembling, dyspnoea, feeling of choking, chest pain/discomfort, nausea/abdominal discomfort, dizziness, paraesthesias, chills and hot flushes, derealization (the experience of the world or people in it seeming lifeless), depersonalization (being detached from oneself) and fear of losing control, 'going crazy' or dying. Typically, the duration of a PA is only a few minutes. A complication is the development of 'anticipatory fear' of the ramifications of having a PA, with the result that the individual may be reluctant to be alone in a public place or away from home. Both current classificatory systems (DSM-IV-TR; ICD-10) stipulate at least three PAs in a 3-

week period where there is no discernable objective danger to the individual, who must be free of anxiety between the discrete PAs. Of the population, around 1% have panic disorder; women are affected more than men and the typical age at onset is 25–44 years. Panic disorder shows familial transmission which is unrelated to GAD. Sodium lactate infusion and breathing carbon dioxide induce PA in susceptible individuals. Selective serotonin reuptake inhibitors (SSRIs), exposure and cognitive–behaviour therapy (CBT) (see Chapter 32) and breathing exercises are the treatments with the strongest evidence base. Other treatments include serotonin and noradrenaline reuptake inhibitors (SNRIs), tricyclic antidepressants (TCAs), reversible monoamine oxidase inhibitors (RIMAs), monoamine oxidase inhibitors (MAOIs), reboxetine and benzodiazepines (NB. tolerance, addiction).

Phobic disorders

Agoraphobia (also known as phobic anxiety/depersonalization), accounts for 60% of phobic patients seen by psychiatrists (66% female, age at onset 15–35 years). Agoraphobia often occurs concurrently with panic disorder and is characterized by anxiety about being in places or situations from which escape might be difficult or in which help may not be available in the event of having a situationally predisposed PA (e.g. being outside home alone, in a crowd, out shopping, on a bridge, in a bus, train or car). The PA-inducing situations are avoided or the presence of a companion is secured.

Generalized anxiety disorders (GAD)

This is characterized by generalized, persistent, excessive anxiety or worry (apprehensive expectation) about a number of events (e.g. work, school performance) which the individual finds difficult to control, lasting for more than 6 months. The anxiety is usually associated with subjective apprehension (fears, worries), increased vigilance, feeling restless and on edge, sleeping difficulties (initial/middle insomnia, fatigue on waking), motor tension (tremor, hyperactive deep reflexes) and autonomic hyperactivity (tachycardia, tachypnoea, dilated pupils). GAD often runs a prolonged, waxing and waning course. Men and individuals with premorbid stability do better. It frequently occurs comorbidly with other anxiety disorders, depression and alcohol and drug abuse. GAD occurs in 2–4% of the general population. It usually begins in early adult life, and affects women more than men. Aetiological factors include a genetic predisposition, childhood experiences

characterized by separations, demands for high achievement and excess conformity, current stressful life events and biological factors (dysfunction of autonomic nervous system reflecting increased sympathetic tone or parasympathetic abnormalities). Several psychophysiological measures are increased in GAD including pulse, skin conduction, forearm blood flow and muscular tension (measured by an electromyogram [EMG]). On the electroencephalograph (EEG), the alpha rhythm is decreased.

Differential diagnosis includes withdrawal from drugs and/or alcohol, excessive caffeine ingestion, depression, schizophrenia and organic causes such as thyrotoxicosis, parathyroid disease, hypoglycaemia, phaeochromocytoma and carcinoid syndrome.

SSRI and SNRI antidepressant treatments as well as buspirone are well supported in clinical trials. Psychological treatments include reassurance, counselling and psychotherapy. Specific psychotherapeutic approaches include CBT (identify morbid anticipatory thoughts and replace with realistic cognitions), insight orientated therapy (explore conflicts) and anxiety management (distraction techniques, breathing and relaxation exercises). Other treatments used include short-term judicious use of benzodiazepines (NB. tolerance, addiction) and beta-blockers (e.g. propanolol), although these are largely indicated for symptomatic relief only.

Social anxiety disorders

Social anxiety disorders are increasingly seen as both common and treatable. They occur more frequently in women. Onset is usually after puberty but often not presenting for medical attention for many years. They result in a marked persistent fear of social performance situations in which the individual is exposed to unfamiliar people or to possible scrutiny by others, and fears that he/she will act in a way that will be humiliating or embarrassing (e.g. blushing, shaking, vomiting). It is probably not a homogeneous clinical entity. Treatment includes drug treatments, notably SSRIs, SNRIs, RIMAs, and MAOIs, behavioural techniques (exposure by systematic desensitization, or modelling) and psychotherapy, which may be supportive (to ensure readjustment of lifestyle) or psychodynamic (exploring conflicts, secondary gain, family approaches).

Specific phobias

Specific phobias (17% of phobic patients seen by psychiatrists; female and male prevalence equal) include fear induced by the presence or anticipation of a specific object or situation (e.g. flying, heights, animals, seeing blood).

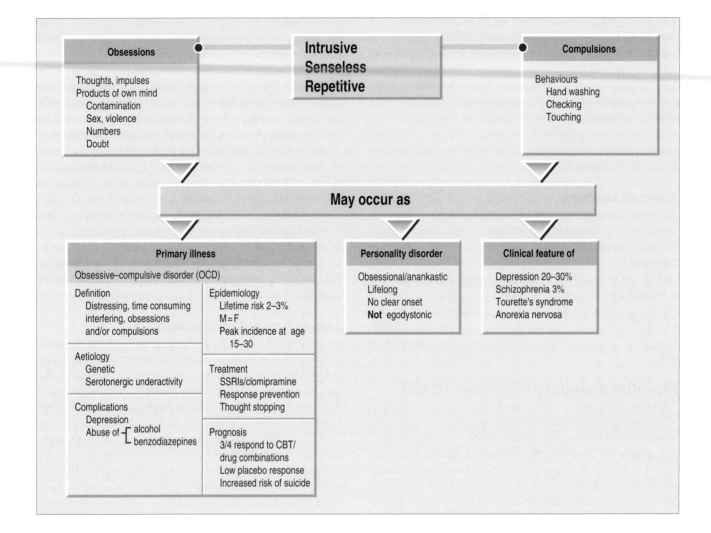

Definition

Obsessions are unwelcome, persistent, recurrent ideas, thoughts, impulses or images which are intrusive, senseless and uncomfortable for the individual, who attempts to suppress or neutralize them and recognizes them as absurd (egodystonic) and a product of his/her own mind. Common obsessions include unpleasant thoughts of blasphemy, sex, violence, contamination, numbers and doubt. Obsessions may take the form of thoughts, images (vivid, morbid or violent scenes), ruminations (continuous pondering) and doubts. Rarer obsessions include arithmomania (counting), onomatomania (the desire to utter a forbidden word) and *folie du pourquoi* (the irresistible habit of seeking explanations for commonplace facts by asking perpetual questions). Obsessions should be distinguished from impulses (thoughts that are not displeasurable [egosyntonic]) and rituals (actions that have a magical quality and are culturally sanctioned).

Compulsions are repetitive, purposeful behaviours performed with reluctance in response to an obsession according to certain rules in a stereotyped fashion, and designed to neutralize or prevent discomfort or a dreaded event. The activity is excessive and not connected to the thought (obsession) in a realistic way. The individual realizes that this egodystonic behaviour is unreasonable. Common compulsions include hand washing, cleaning, counting, checking, touching and constant rearrangement of objects to achieve symmetry.

If resistance to the obsessions or compulsions is attempted, anxiety usually increases until the compulsive activity is performed.

Mild obsessions and compulsions are common in the general population. More severe obsessions and compulsions are prominent symptoms in primary obsessive–compulsive disorder (OCD), are common in depression, schizophrenia and Tourette's syndrome (TS) and may occur in puerperal illness (fear of harming baby), anorexia nervosa, generalized anxiety disorder, dementia, temporal lobe epilepsy, Parkinson's disease, Sydenham's chorea (chorea associated with rheumatic fever), head injury and manganese poisoning.

Anankastic personality disorder

Characteristic features include rigidity of thinking, perfectionism, orderliness, moralistic preoccupation with rules, excessive cleanliness and a tendency to hoard. These are egosyntonic life traits with no obvious onset. The perfectionism may interfere with the affected subject's ability to complete tasks and objectively high standards are seldom achieved. Subjects are often emotionally cold.

Obsessive–compulsive disorder (OCD)
Clinical characteristics
OCD is characterized by egodystonic, time-consuming (>1 hour/day) obsessions and compulsions that interfere with the individual's everyday functioning. Avoidance of stimuli or activities that trigger obsessive–compulsive symptoms is very common. Resistance is characteristic but may not persist. Onset is usually during adolescence. The commonest obsessions are concerned with contamination (43%); hand washing is found in most studies to be the commonest compulsion (85%). Complications include depression and abuse of anxiolytics or alcohol. Severe OCD can lead to as much distress and functional impairment as psychotic illness.

Epidemiology
The epidemiological catchment area (ECA) studies suggest a lifetime prevalence of 1.9–3.2%. Men and women are affected equally.

Aetiology
Causal theories of OCD have changed considerably in the last 30 years. Psychoanalytic theory postulated it to represent a defence against cruel and aggressive fantasies: filling the mind with obsessional thoughts prevents undesirable ideas from entering consciousness. It was also thought to be a defensive regression to a pregenital anal–erotic stage of development. Behaviourists proposed that compulsive behaviour was learned and maintained by operant conditioning processes, the anxiety reduction following the compulsive behaviour strengthening it. More recently, biological factors have been emphasized. In many patients there are genetic influences with a positive family history of OCD (in 50% of cases), tics or TS. It is increasingly accepted that the interaction between behaviour and the environment and on individual patterns of information processing are crucial.

It is thought that there are three types of OCD: (i) genetic and breeding true; (ii) genetic and related to tics or TS; (iii) non-familial. This typology is not universally accepted. Biochemical abnormalities (especially involving serotonin) are now thought to be important in the pathophysiology of OCD. Brain neuroimaging techniques have shown functional abnormalities in the frontal cortex and basal ganglia.

Management
Traditionally, cognitive–behaviour therapy (CBT) has been the mainstay of treatment of OCD, but pharmacological therapy has become increasingly important. CBT includes exposure followed by response prevention for compulsions, and habituation training for obsessions. During exposure and response prevention, the patient is instructed to desist from performing the unwanted compulsive behaviour (e.g. repeated hand washing) while simultaneously being exposed to a situation (e.g. wiping a lavatory seat) likely to increase the need to perform it. Habituation training involves repeated exposure to obsessional thoughts (e.g. the patient listens to a cassette tape continuously repeating out loud his/her obsessional thoughts) without allowing them to be neutralized until the individual habituates and the anxiety decreases. The opposite to habituation training is thought stopping (well known but less effective), during which the patient is encouraged to relax and ruminate until the obsessions are uppermost in his/her mind. The therapist then shouts 'Stop!' and the patient tries to stop ruminating. Drug treatment is with antidepressants which act specifically on serotonin, such as clomipramine and selective serotonin reuptake inhibitors (SSRIs). These drugs are effective even in the absence of coexistent depressive symptomatology. It is now generally agreed that the combination of CBT and medication is the best treatment for OCD. Neuroimaging studies show similar changes in the caudate nucleus in response to CBT and to SSRIs. Overall response to CBT and/or drugs is about 75%; in contrast, placebo responses in clinical trials are very low (5%). The augmentation of an SSRI by antipsychotics may be useful in the treatment of both obsessions and compulsions. Psychosurgery (cingulotomy) is rarely used but may be effective in the most severe and treatment-resistant cases. Deep brain stimulation (DBS) has been used successfully.

Course and prognosis
OCD is chronic with waxing and waning of symptoms. Patients with compulsions only and those with severe symptoms, persistent life stresses or premorbid obsessional personality fare worst. Traditionally, OCD was thought to carry a low risk of suicide; recently, however, the suicide rate (particularly in subjects with coexistent depressive illness) has been found to be considerable.

Anorexia nervosa (AN)		Bulimia nervosa (BN)
Fear of fatness, inflated body image, deliberate weight loss, amenorrhoea, BMI < 17.5	**Definition**	Uncontrolled binge-eating with purging/vomiting Preoccupation with weight and shape

Symptoms
    Preoccupation with food bingeing, purging, vomiting, fear of sleep and social/sexual contact, lack of concentration, feeling cold, depression
Signs
    Of AN—lanugo, bradycardia, hypotension, cold extremities, bruising
    Of vomiting—see Bulimia
	Clinical features	Fluctuating (normal or excessive) weight
		Signs of vomiting
		    Hypokalaemia, alkalosis, pitted teeth, finger callus, parotid swelling
		Psychiatric
		    Depression, poor impulse control, substance abuse (inc. alcohol)

Onset at age 13–20 (85%) 95% female 1–2% prevalence in female students ↑in higher social class	**Epidemiology**	Onset usually at age 15–30 Prevalence 1–3% Sex ratio 50F : 1M (now increasing in males)
Organic: diabetes (which may coexist with AN), Addison's, malabsorption, malignancy (all unlikely) Psychotic: schizophrenia (delusions *re* food)	**Differential diagnosis**	Psychiatric: AN Neurological: Kleine–Levin, Kluver–Bucy

Genetic—family history of eating disorders, OCD, obsessional personality
High conflict, enmeshed family interaction
Cultural and peer-group pressure to diet
	Aetiology	Dietary restraint triggers binge/starve cycle
		Female excess due to
		    Socio-cultural pressures
		    ↑diet-induced serotonin hypofunction

Medical stabilization
Family interventions
Motivational counselling
CBT/IPT
Hospitalization if
    Weight loss severe/rapid
    Signficant physical abnormalities
Fluoxetive may aid weight gain
	Management	Medical stabilization
		CBT/IPT
		SSRIs (less effective than CBT)

40% recovery
35% improvement
20% chronicity
5% mortality
Long-term risk of osteoporosis
	Prognosis	Poor if
		    Low BMI
		    High frequency of purging
		30–40% remission with CBT/IPT

Anorexia nervosa (AN)

AN is characterized by a morbid fear of fatness, deliberate weight loss, distorted body image, amenorrhoea and a body mass index (BMI—defined as weight [kg]/ht [m]^2) of less than 17.5.

Associated features include preoccupation with food (dieting, often with specific fat and carbohydrate avoidance, and sometimes preparation of elaborate meals for others), hyperactivity (with vigorous exercise to lose weight), constipation, cold intolerance, social isolation, body disparagement, fear of sexuality, depressive symptoms and obsessive–compulsive (often perfectionistic) phenomena. Self-consciousness about eating in public and social isolation is often found. Sufferers usually fall into 'restrictive' (minimal food intake and exercise) or 'bulimic' (episodic binge eating with laxative use and induced vomiting) subtypes. Emaciation is often disguised by make-up and baggy clothes. The skin is usually dry and yellow and the trunk and face covered in fine 'lanugo' hair.

Bradycardia, hypotension, anaemia, leucopenia and osteoporosis are common. Consequences of repeated vomiting include hypokalaemia, alkalosis, pitted teeth, parotid swelling and scarring of the dorsum of the hand.

Ninety-five per cent are women; 85% have an onset at age 13–20 years. AN is increasingly seen in children, where the sex ratio is nearly equal. AN in men has a later onset (typically 17–24 years). Prevalence rates of about 1–2% in schoolgirls and female university students have been reported. Higher rates are found in higher socio-economic classes.

Aetiological factors include precipitation by the physical and psychological changes of adolescence and by stress. A genetic component is indicated by the higher concordance for AN in monozygotic (60%) than dizygotic (10%) twins, and the high positive family history of eating disorders, obsessive–compulsive disorders and obsessional personality. Desire to avoid the consequences of sexual maturity has been implicated. Family difficulties are effects rather than causes of the AN.

Differential diagnosis includes organic causes of low weight (e.g. diabetes mellitus), which are not usually associated with abnormal attitudes to weight or eating. Diabetes may coexist with AN. Psychiatric causes of low weight include depression (which may also coexist with AN), psychotic disorders with delusions concerning food, and substance or alcohol abuse. There is an important overlap between AN and bulimia nervosa.

Management initially involves medical stabilization and exclusion of other diagnoses. Coexistent depression should improve with weight gain even without antidepressants. Individuals with AN value their emaciated state and typically are ambivalent about treatment. A good therapeutic relationship and motivational counselling are important elements in AN management. For adolescents with AN, family interventions focused on the eating disorder are the treatment of choice. For adult patients with AN (who have a longer duration and previous failed treatments) a range of specific psychological therapies are effective, including cognitive–behaviour therapy (CBT), interpersonal psychotherapy (IPT), focal psychodynamic therapy and family therapy. Hospitalization (sometimes compulsory) may be necessary if weight loss is severe and rapid, if suicide risk is significant or if there are significant physical abnormalities resulting from starvation or purging. At BMI < 13.5 risk of death from fatal arrhythmia or hypoglycaemia is high and in-patient treatment is indicated. In very severe cases, nasogastric feeding may be instigated without the patient's consent under the provisions of the Mental Health Act.

Specialist in-patient programmes typically provide a structured symptom-focused treatment regime to achieve weight restoration. Behavioural reward systems were used to achieve weight gain during in-patient treatment, but are now widely regarded as punitive and obsolete. Throughout in-patient refeeding, the patient's physical state needs careful monitoring. Drugs which speed gastric emptying (metoclopramide) may reduce bloating and facilitate refeeding. Fluoxetine may be helpful in maintaining weight gain.

Prognosis is variable. About 40% of people recover completely, 35% improve, 20% develop a chronic eating disorder and 5% die from AN. Osteoporosis is a long-term complication.

Bulimia nervosa (BN)

The core feature of BN is binge eating (20 000 kcal in a session) with a sense of loss of control, and compensatory vomiting and/or purging. Dieting, fasting, laxatives and diuretics are also often used. Preoccupation with body weight and shape is also crucial.

Binge eating disorder (BED) without compensatory behaviours typically leads to obesity.

Clinical features include normal or excessive weight (which often fluctuates), and stigmata of excessive vomiting. Sufferers may describe a trance-like state during bingeing. Amenorrhoea occurs in 50% (despite normal weight). Hypokalaemia may lead to dysrhythmias or to renal damage; acute oesophageal tears can occur during forced vomiting. Psychiatric features include intense self-loathing and associated depression. In 'multi-impulsive bulimia' alcohol and drug misuse, deliberate self-harm, stealing and sexual disinhibition coexist. Poor impulse control seems to be the common pathology.

Binge eating is common in adolescence; the prevalence of true BN is 1–3%, with a 50:1 female preponderance. Presentation is later than for AN (late teens or 20s), although onset is often earlier.

Aetiological features include dietary restraint (to which women are more socio-culturally prone) triggering a binge–starve cycle which may in turn reduce serotonergic tone. There is an excess of alcohol and substance abuse, depression and BN in first-degree relatives.

Differential diagnosis must consider AN, affective disorder and obesity. Rare neurological causes of overeating include Kleine–Levin (associated hypersomnia) and Klüver–Bucy (compulsive orality and hypersexuality) syndromes. Diabetic women with BN may omit insulin to lose weight.

Management involves medical stabilization and psychotherapy (usually CBT or IPT; see Chapter 32) to establish a regular eating programme, re-establish control of diet and address underlying abnormal cognitions. Antidepressants have an independent antibulimic effect, best established for fluoxetine (60 mg), but are less effective than CBT.

Prognosis is poor in patients with a low BMI and a high frequency of purging. The short-term benefits of treatment are, however, reasonably well established, with CBT or IPT giving about 30–40% remission.

Obesity

This is defined as a BMI >30. Its prevalence is culturally variable (high in the USA). Mild to moderate (but not severe) obesity is commoner in women and with increasing age. Aetiological factors include weight-controlling genes (e.g. leptins), family and cultural norms, high availability of cheap calorific foods and a sedentary life style. Management involves a behavioural and educational programme to re-establish sensible eating, and cognitive and/or supportive psychotherapy addressing secondary low self-esteem. Anti-obesity medications such as sibutramine or orlistat are only of short-term benefit. Surgical treatment (jaw wiring, gastric banding, resection or bypass) is indicated in severe refractory cases.

Pica

Pica is defined as the persistent eating of non-nutritive substances (e.g. coal or soil). It is normal in very young children; mild forms are often seen in pregnancy. Its persistence may reflect underlying nutritional deficiency or psychiatric illness: particularly learning disability, autism or schizophrenia. Management involves treatment of underlying conditions and behavioural modification.

Disorders of personality

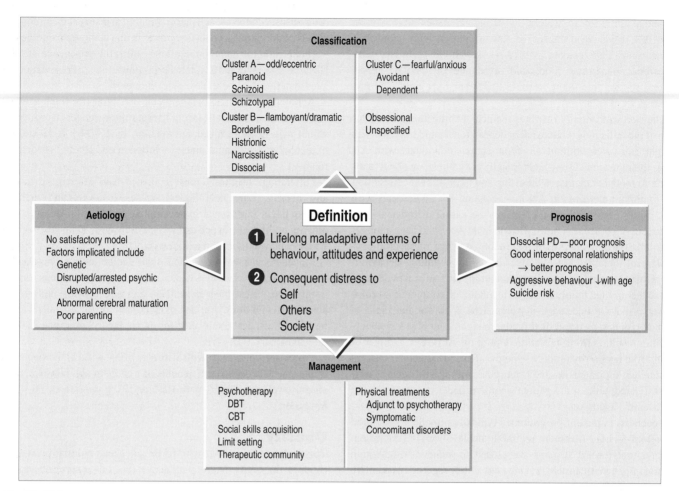

Classification

Cluster A—odd/eccentric
  Paranoid
  Schizoid
  Schizotypal
Cluster B—flamboyant/dramatic
  Borderline
  Histrionic
  Narcissitic
  Dissocial

Cluster C—fearful/anxious
  Avoidant
  Dependent

Obsessional
Unspecified

Aetiology

No satisfactory model
Factors implicated include
  Genetic
  Disrupted/arrested psychic
    development
  Abnormal cerebral maturation
  Poor parenting

Definition

1. Lifelong maladaptive patterns of behaviour, attitudes and experience
2. Consequent distress to
  Self
  Others
  Society

Prognosis

Dissocial PD—poor prognosis
Good interpersonal relationships
  → better prognosis
Aggressive behaviour ↓with age
Suicide risk

Management

Psychotherapy
  DBT
  CBT
Social skills acquisition
Limit setting
Therapeutic community

Physical treatments
  Adjunct to psychotherapy
  Symptomatic
  Concomitant disorders

Definition

Both ICD-10 and DSM-IV-TR define personality disorders (PDs) as persistent, lifelong, deeply ingrained maladaptive patterns of inner experience and behaviour that characterize the individual, deviating markedly from the expectations of his/her culture. Such patterns are not infrequently also manifest early in the individual's development and persist into adulthood. They are frequently associated with subjective/personal distress and/or have adverse effects on interpersonal relations and/or society. PDs are characterized by problems in cognition (ways of perceiving and interpreting self, others, events), affectivity (range, intensity, appropriateness of affective response), interpersonal functioning, impulse control and occupational and social performance.

Assessment of personality

Personality assessments include self-report measures such as the Personality Diagnostic Questionnaire (PDQ) and structured interviews (e.g. Structured Clinical Interview for Personality Disorders [SCID]; Personality Assessment Schedule [PAS]).

Epidemiology

Ten per cent of the adult population have a PD of at least mild severity, as do 20% of general practitioner (GP) attenders, 30% of

psychiatric out-patients and 40% of psychiatric in-patients. The prevalence of some subcategories decreases with age.

Aetiology

There is no single satisfactory aetiological model for PD. Factors implicated include genetic influences (monozygotic/dizygotic concordance; XYY individuals display increased criminality irrespective of IQ or socio-economic class). Psychodynamic theories suggest that PDs result from disrupted/arrested psychic development (e.g. defective and infantile ego functions; defective object relations). Adverse intrauterine, perinatal or postnatal factors leading to abnormal cerebral maturation may predispose to PD, as may poor parenting and social reinforcement of abnormal behaviours. An underactive autonomic nervous system has been implicated in dissocial PD. As a rule of thumb, 'genes' and 'environment' contribute approximately equally to the total pool of personality traits.

Classification and characteristics

The clinical characteristics of specific PDs, grouped (following DSM-IV-TR) into three clusters, are summarized below. It should be noted that patients (particularly those with severe PD) may fulfil the criteria for more than one PD diagnosis.

Cluster 'A' (odd/eccentric)

1 *Paranoid PD*: cold affect, pervasive distrust, suspiciousness of others, preoccupation with doubts about the fidelity or trustworthiness of friends/spouse, reluctance to confide, bearing grudges, reading negative meanings into remarks, hypersensitivity to rebuffs and a grandiose sense of personal rights.

2 *Schizoid PD*: social withdrawal, a restricted range of emotional expression, little interest in sex, restricted pleasure, lacking confidantes, indifference to praise or criticism, aloofness and insensitivity to social norms.

3 *Schizotypal PD*: pervasive social and interpersonal deficits, ideas of reference, magical thinking, unusual perceptions (e.g. bodily illusions), vague, circumstantial, tangential thinking, suspiciousness, inappropriate/constricted affect, eccentricity and excessive social anxiety. Schizotypal PDs are more common in relatives of people with schizophrenia.

Cluster 'B' (flamboyant/dramatic)

1 *Borderline PD* (impulsive): unstable and intense interpersonal relationships, self-image and affect, self-damaging impulsivity (spending, sex, substance abuse, reckless driving, binge eating), identity confusion, chronic anhedonia, recurrent suicidal or self-mutilating behaviour, transient paranoid ideation and frantic efforts to avoid real or imagined abandonment.

2 *Histrionic PD*: excessive shallow emotionality, attention seeking, suggestibility, shallow/labile affect, inappropriate sexual seductiveness but frigidity and immaturity, narcissism, grandiosity, exploitative actions.

3 *Narcissitistic PD*: pervasive grandiosity, lack of empathy and hypersensitivity to the evaluation of others.

4 *Dissocial PD* (antisocial; psychopathic; sociopathic): persistent disregard for the rights or safety of others, gross irresponsibility, incapacity for maintaining relationships, irritability, low frustration tolerance and aggressive threshold, incapacity to experience guilt or profit from experience, deceitfulness, impulsivity, disregard for personal safety, proneness to blame others. Dissocial PD is important legally; in some countries (e.g. UK) it can justify detention under the Mental Health Act (see Chapter 28).

Cluster 'C' (fearful/anxious)

1 *Avoidant PD* (anxious): persistent feelings of tension and inadequacy, social inhibition, unwillingness to become involved with people unless certain of being liked and restriction in lifestyle to maintain physical security.

2 *Dependent PD* (asthenic): an excessive need to be taken care of leading to submissive and clinging behaviour, fears of separation, difficulty in making everyday decisions without excessive advice, needing others to assume responsibility, difficulty in expressing disagreement for fear of loss of support/approval, difficulty in initiating projects (because of lack of self-confidence), going to lengths to gain support from others, constantly needing close relationships, undue compliance with other's wishes, unwilling to make demands on people and preoccupation with fears of being left alone.

Other PDs include *obsessional* (anankastic; see Chapter 10) and *unspecified*.

Management

Successful management depends on securing an adequate treatment alliance so that the patient is able to work together with a therapist. Deep-seated mistrust and ambivalence therefore need to be addressed early in treatment, and the long-term and arduous nature of treatment should be discussed with the patient at the outset. Multidisciplinary and multi-agency work is often required. Admission to hospital, day hospital care or intensive community care during periods of crisis may be necessary.

Specific therapeutic techniques include a range of psychological techniques, particularly individual and group supportive therapies, cognitive–behaviour therapy (CBT) and, specifically for borderline PD, dialectical behaviour therapy (DBT) (see Chapter 32). Limit-setting and confrontation, together with pro-social skills acquisition are important adjuncts. Physical treatments have not been adequately evaluated but are useful in treating coexisting conditions (e.g. depression) and in the management of acute subjective distress, particularly in an out-patient setting where management may need to focus on symptom suppression, especially in relation to impulsivity and aggression. Drug treatment is most effective if it is individually-tailored and symptom focused. Antipsychotics may be useful for cognitive symptoms (e.g. ideas of reference, depersonalization), impulsivity and intense angry affect. Monoamine oxidase inhibitors (MAOIs) may be helpful in some borderline PDs, alleviating the abnormal mood (empty, lonely, bored). Carbamazepine and lithium may help some individuals with episodic behavioural dyscontrol and aggression, even in the absence of epileptic, affective or organic features. Drug treatment and psychotherapy in PD are not mutually exclusive and their combination may be summative.

Prognosis

In general, individuals with PDs show decreased aggressive behaviour with age, although the ability to form successful interpersonal relationships remains poor. Borderline PD carries a relatively favourable prognosis, with clinical recovery in over 50% at 10–25-year follow-up; schizoid and schizotypal patients tend to remain isolated. Dissocial PD carries a particularly poor prognosis. Certain individuals with PDs may relieve subjective discomfort by abusing alcohol and psychoactive substances, resulting in dependence. There is an increased risk of suicide in people with PDs; between 30% and 60% of completed suicides have evidence of PD.

Obsessional PDs are at high risk of progression to obsessive–compulsive disorder (OCD; see Chapter 10) or to depression; paranoid and schizotypal PD may progress to schizophrenia. In contrast, schizoid PD does not predispose to schizophrenia. Some PDs may confer susceptibility to physical illness (e.g. obsessional PD and duodenal ulcer).

Cluster B subcategories may represent the purest of the three DSM clusters in terms of a natural history of 'breeding true'. The severity of PD is also influential in the prognosis, although there is no general agreement in how to measure it reliably. One potential measure relates to the 'breadth' of PD pathology as rated by the number of PD symptoms and signs, for example, as measured by the total score on PDQ (see above). An alternative is to identify as 'severe' those who have subcategories of PD from more than one of the three DSM clusters, since some PD individuals have many subcategories, i.e. PD comorbidity.

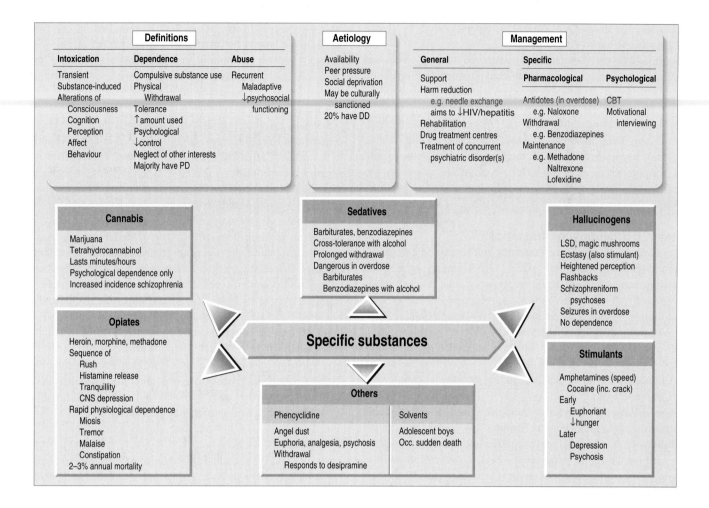

Acute intoxication refers to transient disturbances of consciousness, cognition, perception, affect or behaviour following the administration of a psychoactive substance (PS). **Harmful** PS use implies damage to the individual's health and adverse effects on family and society.

Dependence involves physiological and/or psychological elements. The former include a withdrawal state, tolerance (increasing doses of PSs needed for the same effect) and the PS being taken in larger amounts or for longer than intended. Psychological dependence involves a sense of compulsion to take the PS, difficulties in controlling PS use, increasing time spent obtaining, ingesting or recovering from the PS, persistence with PS use despite awareness of harmful consequences and the persistent but futile wish to cut down PS use. There may also be reduction in important social, occupational or recreational activities because of PS use.

Substance abuse (persistent and sporadic excessive PS use leading to significant impairment or distress) may involve failure to fulfil obligations at work/school/home, hazardous behaviour (e.g. driving) and legal problems (e.g. arrests).

Aetiology and management

Socio-environmental factors (availability, peer pressure, depriva-

tion, abuse) are key determinants of PS use. Neurobiological mechanisms, pre-existing psychopathology (e.g. attention–deficit disorder rendering an individual vulnerable to cocaine use), personality disorders (borderline or antisocial), iatrogenic factors (e.g. prescribed benzodiazepines [BDZs]), conditioned learning and the pharmacological properties of the PS may all contribute. The majority of PS misusers have personality disorders (PD). At least 20% have other psychiatric disorders (comorbidity/dual diagnosis [DD]), which may include substance-induced (e.g amphetamine, cocaine) psychoses and expected effects of intoxication or withdrawal. Management of DD patients should involve an integrated approach with a multidisciplinary team trained in the management of both sets of disorders, which should be treated concurrently. The use of certain PSs is socially/culturally sanctioned (e.g. opium and Khat).

As well as being obtained illicitly, PSs may be obtained from doctors (ostensibly therapeutically). Some may legally be bought from chemists (codeine) or shops (solvents). In the UK, some PSs (heroin, morphine, cocaine, cannabis, amphetamines, barbiturates and lysergic acid diethylamide [LSD]) are controlled under the **Misuse of Drugs Act**, rendering supply, possession, production, import or export illegal without appropriate licensing. Both in the

UK and the USA, polysubstance abuse has increased. Management involves general support (residential rehabilitation and aftercare; drug treatment units), specific antidotes in overdose (e.g. naloxone), medication to minimize withdrawal symptoms (e.g. BDZs) and long-term medication (e.g. methadone replacement for opiates or naltrexone to neutralize opiate effects). Cognitive–behaviour therapy (CBT) and related psychological approaches, such as motivational interviewing self-help groups, are also used. Infection (human immunodeficiency virus [HIV] and hepatitis—especially C) is now recognized as the greatest risk associated with injected drug use. Management strategies (harm reduction) are increasingly targeted at infection risk minimization (e.g. needle exchange).

Specific substances
Opiates

Opiates include *heroin*, *morphine*, *methadone* and dextramoromide. They may be smoked (chasing the dragon), sniffed (snorting), taken orally, intravenously (mainlining), intramuscularly or subcutaneously (skin popping). After an intensely pleasurable 'buzz' or 'rush', and release of histamine (itching, reddening of eyes), a sense of peace and detachment occurs, succeeded by central nervous system (CNS) depression. Tolerance and withdrawal develop quickly. Ten per cent of opiate misusers become dependent but only 10% of these ever seek help; 2–3% die annually. Of the remainder, 25% are abstinent at 5 years and 40% at 10 years. Miosis, tremor, malaise, apathy, constipation, weakness, impotence, neglect, malnutrition and evidence of HIV and other infection (hepatitis C) are signs of chronic dependence. Early withdrawal symptoms (24–48 hours) include craving, flu-like symptoms, sweating and yawning. Mydriasis, abdominal cramps, diarrhoea, agitation, restlessness, piloerection ('gooseflesh') and tachycardia occur later (7–10 days). Symptoms may be controlled by symptomatic treatment or with methadone (less euphoriant, relatively long half-life and used for long-term maintenance)—lofexidine is used for detoxification, naltrexone for relapse prevention and buprenorphine for detoxification and replacement. Signs of overdose (often accidental) include miosis and respiratory depression and may require naloxone.

Hallucinogens

Hallucinogens include *LSD*, which produces psychological (e.g. perceptions heightened) and physiological (pupils dilated, peripheral vasoconstriction, increased temperature) effects, but not dependence. Adverse effects include 'flashbacks' (visual, occurring spontaneously for up to 1 year), schizophreniform psychoses and (in overdose) seizures. *Ecstasy* (MDMA), a synthetic amphetamine analogue, has mixed stimulant and hallucinogenic effects and can induce hyperactivity and potentially fatal dehydration and hyperpyrexia. *Magic mushrooms* (Psylocybin) have effects similar to but are less intense than LSD.

Stimulants

Amphetamines (speed) taken orally or intravenously, cause euphoria, increased concentration and energy, mydriasis, tachycardia and hyperreflexia followed by depression, fatigue and headache. Acute use may induce a schizophreniform psychosis. *Cocaine* may be sniffed chewed or injected intravenously. Its effects (restlessness, increased energy, abolition of fatigue and hunger) resemble hypomania and lasts 20 minutes. Visual/tactile hallucinations of insects (formication) and paranoid psychoses occur. Post-cocaine dysphoria ('the crash'), with sleeplessness and intense depression, precedes withdrawal (depression, insomnia and craving). 'Crack' (a purified very addictive form of cocaine) is smoked. The crack 'high' is extremely short and withdrawal persecutory delusions are common.

Cannabis

The active compound of *marijuana* (pot, grass, hashish, ganja) is tetrahydrocannabinol. The effects are psychological (euphoria, relaxation, well-being, omnipotence, hallucinations) and physiological (increased appetite, lowered body temperature). Substantial psychological dependence occurs. Adverse effects include conjunctival irritation, decreased spermatogenesis, lung disease, flashbacks, transient psychoses and apathy. Cannabis use is associated with increased incidence of schizophrenia.

Sedatives and hypnotics

Barbiturates (now rarely used) produce relaxation and sedation, and induce tolerance and dependence with withdrawal anxiety, tremor, insomnia and convulsions. Overdose may cause respiratory depression. Withdrawal is treated with BDZs or anticonvulsants. *BDZs* produce dependence, withdrawal (which may mimic the problem for which they were prescribed or manifest with delerium and/or seizures) and tolerance. BDZ dependence is often iatrogenic, although BDZs are also common street drugs.

Others

Solvents are typically sniffed experimentally by groups of boys (8–19 years). Initial euphoria is followed by drowsiness. Psychological dependence is common but physical dependence is rare. Chronic abuse results in weight loss, nausea, vomiting, arrythmias, bronchospasm and cognitive impairment. Toxic effects (sometimes fatal) include hepatorenal or cerebral damage, aplastic anaemia and polyneuropathy. *Phencyclidine* (PCP; 'Angel Dust') is usually smoked. Effects include euphoria and peripheral analgesia and impaired consciousness or psychosis which may require antipsychotics.

14 Alcohol abuse and dependence

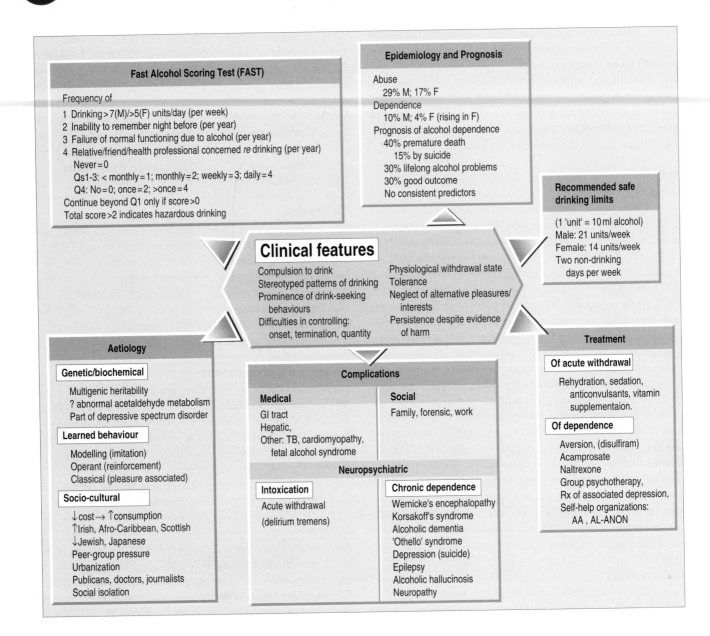

Fast Alcohol Scoring Test (FAST)

Frequency of
1 Drinking > 7(M)/>5(F) units/day (per week)
2 Inability to remember night before (per year)
3 Failure of normal functioning due to alcohol (per year)
4 Relative/friend/health professional concerned *re* drinking (per year)
    Never = 0
    Qs1-3: < monthly = 1; monthly = 2; weekly = 3; daily = 4
    Q4: No = 0; once = 2; >once = 4
Continue beyond Q1 only if score >0
Total score >2 indicates hazardous drinking

Epidemiology and Prognosis

Abuse
    29% M; 17% F
Dependence
    10% M; 4% F (rising in F)
Prognosis of alcohol dependence
    40% premature death
        15% by suicide
    30% lifelong alcohol problems
    30% good outcome
    No consistent predictors

Recommended safe drinking limits

(1 'unit' = 10 ml alcohol)
Male: 21 units/week
Female: 14 units/week
Two non-drinking
    days per week

Clinical features

Compulsion to drink
Stereotyped patterns of drinking
Prominence of drink-seeking
    behaviours
Difficulties in controlling:
    onset, termination, quantity

Physiological withdrawal state
Tolerance
Neglect of alternative pleasures/
    interests
Persistence despite evidence
    of harm

Aetiology

Genetic/biochemical

Multigenic heritability
? abnormal acetaldehyde metabolism
Part of depressive spectrum disorder

Learned behaviour

Modelling (imitation)
Operant (reinforcement)
Classical (pleasure associated)

Socio-cultural

↓cost → ↑consumption
↑Irish, Afro-Caribbean, Scottish
↓Jewish, Japanese
Peer-group pressure
Urbanization
Publicans, doctors, journalists
Social isolation

Complications

Medical	Social
GI tract	Family, forensic, work
Hepatic,	
Other: TB, cardiomyopathy, fetal alcohol syndrome	

Neuropsychiatric

Intoxication	Chronic dependence
Acute withdrawal	Wernicke's encephalopathy
(delirium tremens)	Korsakoff's syndrome
	Alcoholic dementia
	'Othello' syndrome
	Depression (suicide)
	Epilepsy
	Alcoholic hallucinosis
	Neuropathy

Treatment

Of acute withdrawal

Rehydration, sedation,
    anticonvulsants, vitamin
    supplementaion.

Of dependence

Aversion, (disulfiram)
Acamprosate
Naltrexone
Group psychotherapy,
Rx of associated depression,
Self-help organizations:
    AA , AL-ANON

Definition and clinical features

The term 'alcohol abuse' implies regular or binge consumption of alcohol sufficient to cause physical, neuropsychiatric or social damage. The conventional safe drinking limits are 21 units per week for men and 14 for women (a 'unit' of alcohol [10 mL] representing roughly a small glass of wine, a pub single of spirits, or a half pint of beer), with at least 2 drink-free days each week. Even much smaller amounts may be hazardous to the fetus. 'Alcohol dependence' is a syndrome with cognitive, behavioural and psychological features central to which are the compulsion to drink, preoccupation with alcohol, stereotyped drinking pattern, loss of the ability to regulate drinking, altered tolerance of the intoxicant effects of alcohol (initially increased but dramatically reduced late in the disorder), withdrawal phenomena and persistence even after attempted abstinence.

Epidemiology

Prevalence rates world-wide vary widely, and are related to overall consumption levels, availability and price. In the UK, 29% of men and 17% of women drink more than the safe limits. The prevalence of alcohol dependence is 7.4%, with a male/female ratio of 3 : 1. Rates in women and in adolescents are increasing.

Detection and screening

Neither alcohol abuse nor dependence is always clinically obvious. Their detection is crucial not only to enable appropriate counselling and treatment, and thus avoid long-term complications, but also to avoid acute withdrawal in the context of unplanned abstinence as, for example, after surgery. General practitioners (GPs) and junior hospital staff should have a high index of suspicion in subjects with medical or psychiatric conditions associated with alcohol, and those with two or more drink/driving offences. Many cases can be identified by documenting a 'typical drinking week'. Screening questionnaires are also helpful (see diagram). The CAGE (have you tried to Cut down drinking; have people Annoyed you by suggesting you do so; have you felt Guilty about drinking; have you needed an Eye-opener) remains widely used. The FAST is an improved screening tool designed for busy medical settings. There are four items (see diagram), but for over 50% of people only the first question 'How often do you have eight or more drinks [units] on one occasion?' needs to be asked. The answers 'never' or 'less than monthly' indicate that problem drinking is unlikely. Additional informant history can be revealing. Physical examination may reveal alcoholic stigmata, particularly signs of liver disease (spider naevi, palmar erythema, gynaecomastia) and peripheral neuropathy. Laboratory test results suggestive of problem drinking include macrocytosis without anaemia and raised γ-glutamyl transferase. Carbohydrate defficient transferrin (CDT) indicates recent harmful use, as do high blood or urine ethanol levels without obvious intoxication.

Aetiology

Aetiology is clearly multifactorial. Genetic factors have been implicated in both animal and human studies, and by the striking differences in prevalence of alcohol dependence and abuse in some racial groups (e.g. high in indigenous Americans and Australians, low in Chinese and Japanese). These may be mediated by alterations in alcohol metabolism, those at low risk producing more (hangover-causing) acetaldehyde. Heritability appears multigenic. There is often a positive family history of depression, suggesting that alcohol-related problems may form part of a genetically determined 'depressive spectrum'. Social factors include occupation (high risk in the armed forces, doctors, publicans, journalists); cultural, particularly peer-group, influences (low rates in Jews, high in Scots and Irish) and the cost of alcoholic drinks. Behavioural models stress learning by imitation (modelling), by social reinforcement (operant conditioning) and by classical conditioning (drinking to avoid withdrawal symptoms and the association between drinking and pleasure). Risk increases in the presence of chronic psychiatric or physical illness, particularly if complicated by chronic pain.

Complications

Complications include *acute intoxication*, characterized by slurred speech, impaired coordination and judgment, labile affect and, in severe cases, hypoglycaemia, stupor and coma. Differential diagnosis involves other causes of acute confusion, particularly head trauma. *Acute withdrawal* usually occurs within 1–2 days of abstinence and is characterized by malaise, nausea, autonomic hyperactivity, tremulousness, lability of mood, insomnia and transient hallucinations or illusions (usually visual). Seizures are a recognized complication. Severe withdrawal 'delirium tremens' has a mortality of up to 15%, partly as a result of other *medical complications*. These may be gastrointestinal (gastritis, peptic ulcer, pancreatitis, hepatitis, cirrhosis, oesophageal varices and/or carcinoma), haematological (anaemia, thrombocytopaenia) and cardiovascular (cardiomyopathy, hypertension). The most dramatic *neuropsychiatric complication* is Wernicke's encephalopathy (secondary to thiamine deficiency and characterized by ataxia, nystag-

mus, ophthalmoplegia and acute confusion), which may recover with acute administration of thiamine but may develop if untreated into Korsakoff's psychosis (resolution of acute neurological signs but profound loss of short-term memory). A more generalized dementia may also occur. Other neuropsychiatric complications include peripheral neuropathy, cerebellar degeneration, alcoholic hallucinosis (usually threatening second-person voices in a clear sensorium), pathological or morbid jealousy (see Chapter 36), symptoms of depression and/or anxiety and erectile or ejaculatory impotence. Abuse of other drugs (particularly cross-tolerance with other sedatives such as benzodiazepines) is common. *Social complications* include job loss, marital difficulties, criminal activity or prostitution and alcohol-related road accidents. Alcohol is also often implicated in domestic violence, accidental deaths and homicides. Drinking in pregnancy may harm the fetus (*fetal alcohol syndrome*).

Management

Non-dependent drinkers may respond well to brief interventions, which offer health education and brief advice on reduction of drinking. Management of alcohol dependence needs to consider biological, psychological and social factors, and often requires a coordinated multidisciplinary and long-term approach.

The first step is to achieve abstinence and may require acute 'detoxification' which (like acute withdrawal) involves general support (adequate nutrition, reality orientation, good lighting) and measures to avoid specific complications. The latter include initially high but rapidly tailing sedation (benzodiazepines—such as chlordiazepoxide or diazepam, except in liver disease) to prevent seizures and control hallucinosis (this may also require antipsychotics; haloperidol has little effect on seizure threshold); rehydration and correction of electrolyte disturbance; and B-vitamin supplementation.

Abstinence may be a more realistic long-term aim than controlled drinking. Maintenance (of abstinence or controlled drinking within safe limits) can include psychotherapy, individual or in groups, aiming at sustaining motivation, learning relapse prevention strategies and developing social routines not reliant on alcohol; treatment of coexistent depression and/or anxiety; self-help groups (such as Alcoholics Anonymous [AA]); and disulfiram which blocks alcohol metabolism, inducing acetaldehyde accumulation if alcohol is ingested with resultant flushing, headache, anxiety and nausea. Acamprosate reduces craving and has recently been licensed for the maintenance of abstinence in the detoxified patient; naltrexone has a similar effect.

Prevention involves reducing overall alcohol consumption; measures can include increasing taxation on alcohol and restricting its advertising and/or sale. Health education may also be helpful, although there is not strong evidence for its effectiveness in reducing alcohol consumption.

Prognosis

Alcohol dependence is characterized by periods of remission and relapse; 40% of subjects will die prematurely (15% by suicide) and a further 30% have lifelong alcohol-related problems. About one-third have a favourable outcome, although there are no factors that have been consistently found to identify a good prognosis.

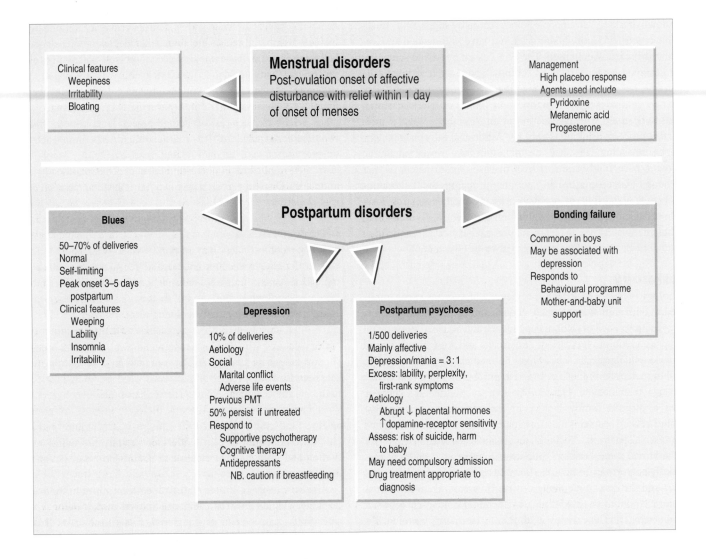

The premenstrual syndrome (PMS)

PMS represents a disturbance of mood, often accompanied by other psychiatric features (insomnia, poor concentration, irritability, poor impulse control, food craving) and/or physical complaints (headache, breast tenderness and bloating). The onset is after ovulation, with rapid relief within 24 hours of the onset of menstrual flow. In DSM-IV-TR it is categorized as Premenstrual Dysphoric Disorder (PDD); in ICD-10 it is listed as a physical disorder. PMS is difficult to measure and prevalence estimates vary widely. Up to 95% of women of reproductive age have some premenstrual symptoms, but only 3–8% meet the criteria for PDD. Diagnosis is clinical by diaries of symptoms and menstruation. There is little evidence that academic performance is impaired by PMS: some studies have shown an excess of criminal activity at the end of the menstrual cycle. Possible aetiological factors include a decrease in serotonin levels after ovulation in affected women, fluctuations in electrolyte and sex hormone levels and consequent neurotransmitter changes. Selective serotonin reuptake inhibitors (SSRIs) have proved particularly beneficial for symptomatic treatment. High placebo response rates have been reported in studies of PMS.

Mental illness during pregnancy

New episodes of severe mental illness and suicide in pregnancy are rare. Significant depression or anxiety occurs in about 10% of women in the first trimester. Those with a past psychiatric history or with conflicting feelings about the pregnancy (such as a past or currently contemplated termination) are at particular risk. Recent evidence suggests that depression may also be common in the third trimester (10–15%). A number of psychiatric drugs are known to have adverse effects on the fetus or newborn. Some (e.g. lithium, benzodiazepines) increase the risk of congenital malformations. Others can affect the newborn child if given in the third trimester (e.g. antipsychotics can induce an extrapyramidal syndrome in the baby and anxiolytics can cause a 'floppy baby syndrome'). Potential benefits of prescribing in individual cases must be weighed up against these risks, but potential risks of not prescribing, such as the impact on the fetus and mother of disturbed behaviour, suicide, and impact on bonding of an untreated depression after birth should also be considered.

Postpartum disorders

These range from the mild, common and transient postpartum blues, through postpartum depression to the rare but florid postpartum psychoses. Risk of postpartum disorders appears similar after perinatal death (and less after abortion) to that after normal pregnancy. Adequate opportunity to grieve should be provided, and bereavement counselling may be required. Formal psychiatric illness following termination of pregnancy is rare, but guilt feelings are common, need ventilating and may re-emerge in subsequent pregnancies. Women who have a history of serious mental illness, postpartum or otherwise, have a risk of recurrence after childbirth of between 1 in 2 and 1 in 3. There is an increased risk of relapse after childbirth in affective disorders and probably also schizophrenia. It is important to ask about psychiatric history at the antenatal clinic so that anticipatory management plans can be made.

Postpartum blues

Postpartum blues occur after 50–70% of deliveries and should not be regarded as abnormal. The symptoms experienced are, however, sufficiently severe and out of the ordinary to warrant attention. The cardinal features are affective, with marked emotional lability, crying without external cause, irritability, sleep disturbance and disproportionate fear of inability to cope with the baby. Onset may be at any time within the first 10 postpartum days but is typically on days 3–5. More rarely, the blues may present (usually on days 1 or 2) with elation and irritability. The aetiology remains unclear; women with a history of severe PMS are at higher risk; elevated antepartum progesterone levels and precipitate postpartum falls in oestrogen, progesterone and sodium have been implicated. No clear relationship with obstetric or social variables has been demonstrated. The blues are self-limiting, usually within a few days. No specific intervention is required (apart from reassurance), although more persistent depression must be excluded. Appropriate antenatal education is helpful.

Postpartum depression

Postpartum depression occurs in 10–15% of new mothers, with onset within the first 6 weeks after delivery. Clinical features are similar to those of depression at other times, though suicidal thoughts are less common, and guilt concerning the baby common. Unlike the blues, postpartum depression persists for a year or more in 50% of cases. Many cases are undetected and screening for depression is an appropriate part of the 6-week postnatal check. Aetiological factors appear to be predominantly social (although a family history of depression, particularly postpartum, is common), with marital conflicts and a lack of confiding relationships particu-

larly implicated. Management involves full social assessment (including possible risk to the baby), and treatment may include marital therapy, individual (supportive or cognitive) psychotherapy and/or antidepressants. Most antidepressants are excreted in breast milk in concentrations approximating those in maternal plasma. Risks to breast-fed babies are slight but must be considered when initiating antidepressants in women keen to continue breastfeeding. Although deliberate self-harm and suicide are less common in pregnancy and the postpartum year than at other times, suicide is the leading cause of maternal death in the UK.

Postpartum psychoses

Postpartum psychoses occur after about one birth in 500, and usually have an abrupt onset within 2–4 weeks after delivery. The excess is more than can be explained as a 'postponement' of such disorders from pregnancy. The clinical presentation is usually affective, the majority depressive but up to one-third with mania. Postpartum onset of schizophrenia is relatively rare, but postpartum affective psychoses are often associated with one or more Schneiderian first-rank symptoms, and are likely to show emotional lability and to be subjectively confused. The excess positive family history of affective disorder is similar to that found in bipolar patients. Risk of postpartum recurrence is at least 1 in 5 after one postpartum (or non-postpartum) episode, and up to 1 in 2 after multiple postpartum episodes. Risk appears highest in primiparae, and after instrumental delivery. Dopamine-receptor supersensitivity has been reported in high-risk subjects who subsequently develop postpartum psychoses. Management must include assessment of suicide risk and of risk to the baby, who may suffer from neglect and/or (where the mother is deluded) inappropriate care, deliberate harm or even infanticide. Treatment usually requires hospitalization, sometimes compulsorily, and where possible, with the baby to a specialist mother-and-baby unit. Drug treatment is as appropriate to the clinical presentation, although antidepressants and neuroleptics must be used with caution (and lithium is contraindicated) in breastfeeding mothers. Electroconvulsive therapy (ECT) has been reported to be particularly effective, irrespective of diagnostic group. Short-term prognosis is excellent, although risk of recurrence is similar to that for non-postpartum affective disorder.

Bonding failure

Bonding failure represents the failure to develop the normally intense emotional mother–baby bond, and may be accompanied by hostility towards the baby. It usually occurs in the context of ambivalence about the pregnancy, adverse life events and/or postpartum depression. Management, which should take place in a mother-and-baby unit, involves treatment of underlying conflicts and a combination of supportive and behavioural (modelling) psychotherapy. Prolonged postnatal depression may also affect later social and cognitive development of the child, particularly in boys, even after resolution of the maternal illness.

16 Functional disorders in old age

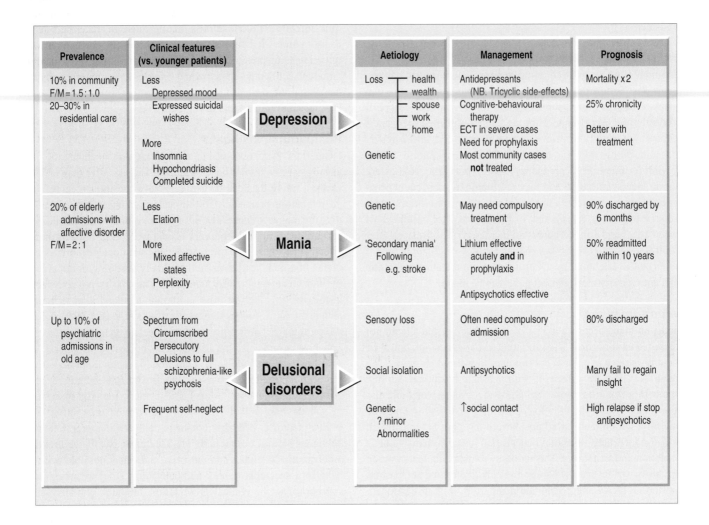

Prevalence	Clinical features (vs. younger patients)		Aetiology	Management	Prognosis
10% in community F/M=1.5:1.0 20–30% in residential care	Less Depressed mood Expressed suicidal wishes	**Depression**	Loss — health — wealth — spouse — work — home Genetic	Antidepressants (NB. Tricyclic side-effects) Cognitive-behavioural therapy ECT in severe cases Need for prophylaxis Most community cases **not** treated	Mortality x2 25% chronicity Better with treatment
	More Insomnia Hypochondriasis Completed suicide				
20% of elderly admissions with affective disorder F/M=2:1	Less Elation	**Mania**	Genetic 'Secondary mania' Following e.g. stroke	May need compulsory treatment Lithium effective acutely **and** in prophylaxis Antipsychotics effective	90% discharged by 6 months 50% readmitted within 10 years
	More Mixed affective states Perplexity				
Up to 10% of psychiatric admissions in old age	Spectrum from Circumscribed Persecutory Delusions to full schizophrenia-like psychosis Frequent self-neglect	**Delusional disorders**	Sensory loss Social isolation Genetic ? minor Abnormalities	Often need compulsory admission Antipsychotics ↑social contact	80% discharged Many fail to regain insight High relapse if stop antipsychotics

Older people suffer from a range of functional psychiatric disorders that may present particular problems in both detection and treatment. The most important of these (depression, mania and the delusional [schizophrenia-like] disorders of late life) are discussed in turn below. Older people are also liable to experience adjustment reactions (particularly bereavement), although the presentation and management of these are essentially the same as earlier in life. In addition, anxiety disorders (both generalized and phobic) are common. General anxiety is often either relatively mild or coexistent with (and responsive to the same treatment approaches as) depression. New phobic disorders, particularly agoraphobia, are often precipitated by traumatic events and frequently persist. Finally, older people may continue to manifest disorders of personality, although the degree of distress and disability they cause usually decreases with increasing age.

Depression in old age
Epidemiology and clinical features
Depression is about as common in late as in middle life. There is good consensus from epidemiological studies that its prevalence in late life is around 13%. Most studies find an over-representation of women (by a factor of about 1.5) and little relationship within the elderly with increasing age. The diagnosis is, however, often 'missed' in older subjects, despite the fact that they frequently consult their doctor; most subjects detected in community surveys have not been treated. This is partly because of the unjustified idea that depression is an inevitable consequence of ageing but also because of important differences in clinical presentation. Depressed mood is less often overt in older depressed subjects, who are also less likely to express suicidal ideation despite being at substantially higher risk of completed suicide. Older depressed subjects are, however, more likely to complain of disturbed sleep, which must be distinguished from the more insidious loss of sleep duration commonly found in normal ageing; to complain of multiple physical problems for which no cause can be found; and to exhibit motor disturbance (retardation and/or agitation). These differences in symptom pattern render conventional diagnostic criteria for depression misleading in old age, since the majority of subjects fulfil

criteria for only 'minor' depression despite similar severity of illness to those with major depression and, paradoxically, a greater proportion with an 'endogenous' pattern of symptoms.

Aetiology

Genetic factors are significant, although the family history is less often positive than in younger depressed patients. In particular, subjects becoming depressed for the first time in late life often have a low genetic loading, but are more likely to have brain-imaging abnormalities, cognitive impairment and poor treatment response. This suggests that late first-onset depression may, in some cases, reflect neurodegenerative change. Vascular risk factors may be particularly important. Social isolation, particularly the lack of confiding relationships, render older people vulnerable to depression, which is often triggered by the experience of loss(es) such as bereavement, deteriorating physical health or financial insecurity. Risk of depression is also high in carers of people with dementia. Being in residential or nursing care doubles the risk of depression in old age.

Management

Both physical and psychological treatments are effective but under-used in older subjects. Reducing social isolation may also be important. Cognitive and behavioural approaches may need to be modified to the needs of an older group but are effective in group as well as individual settings. Tricyclic antidepressants are as effective as in younger subjects, but their utility in practice is diminished by a higher risk of clinically important side-effects, particularly postural hypotension and resultant falls (dangerous, particularly in the presence of age-related osteoporosis which is commoner in women). Newer antidepressants (e.g. selective serotonin reuptake inhibitors [SSRIs], venlafaxine, mirtazapine) may be of particular value in the elderly because of their relative lack of contraindications, safety and favourable side-effect profile. Adherence to antidepressant treatment may be difficult to achieve in older subjects, particularly since they may take longer (up to 8 weeks) to take effect. Electroconvulsive therapy (ECT) is very effective in the more severe depressions of late life, particularly in retarded and/or deluded patients and those refusing food and/or fluid in whom the risk of irreversible physical deterioration is high. Monoamine oxidase inhibitors (MAOIs) and lithium augmentation are effective in some older patients with refractory depression.

Prognosis

Depression in late life carries a mortality rate twice that in matched control subjects. Some of the excess is related to suicide, the risk of which is particularly high in older depressed men. There is also a high risk of chronicity (about 50% if untreated) and of relapse. The prognosis is considerably improved by early detection, with appropriate acute treatment and subsequent prophylaxis; both antidepressants and lithium are effective in preventing depressive relapse.

Mania in old age

Mania in old age was thought rare but in fact accounts for about 20% of all psychiatric admissions for affective disorders in older subjects. Most subjects have a past history of depression; in about 20% the mania is precipitated by acute physical illness such as stroke. Overt elation is less often present than in mania in earlier life, although the patient generally has grandiose ideation, and the clinical picture is more usually of irritability, lability of mood and perplexity—much like that of delirium (see Chapter 17) which is thus the most important differential diagnosis. Antipsychotics are effective in acute treatment, although their prolonged use is to be avoided if possible because of the age-related increase in risk of tardive dyskinesia. Atypical antipsychotics must be used with particular caution (see below). Lithium may be used both acutely and in prophylaxis, although as many as 25% of older subjects (particularly those with Parkinson's disease or dementia) develop neurotoxicity. Both therapeutic and toxic effects of lithium may occur at lower blood levels in old age; close monitoring is therefore necessary. The prognosis with treatment is good, although recurrence occurs in up to 50% by 10 years.

Delusional disorders

These account for 10% of all psychiatric admissions in old age and represents a spectrum of presentations, ranging from highly circumscribed persecutory delusions, through the presence of both delusions and hallucinations to a full-blown schizophrenia-like picture with thought disorder, passivity experiences and/or disorders of possession of thought. The debate as to whether these conditions are distinct from schizophrenia is unresolved. Acute confusional states, delusional depression and early dementia must all be considered in the differential diagnosis. Aetiological factors include a genetic component (with excess family history of psychiatric illness as a whole and particularly schizophrenia), sensory deprivation (particularly deafness) and longstanding social isolation. Brain-imaging abnormalities have been reported. Treatment is often difficult because of lack of insight, but response to antipsychotics, combined if possible with social reintegration, is usually good. As older people are at particular risk of tardive dyskinesia, atypical antipsychotics may be better tolerated. They must however be used with caution in view of the newly recognized risks of stroke and impaired glycaemic control. A substantial minority of patients never regain insight despite good functional recovery. Relapse is frequent if antipsychotics are withdrawn; this must be weighed up against the risk of tardive dyskinesia with their continued use.

17 Acute confusional states (delirium)

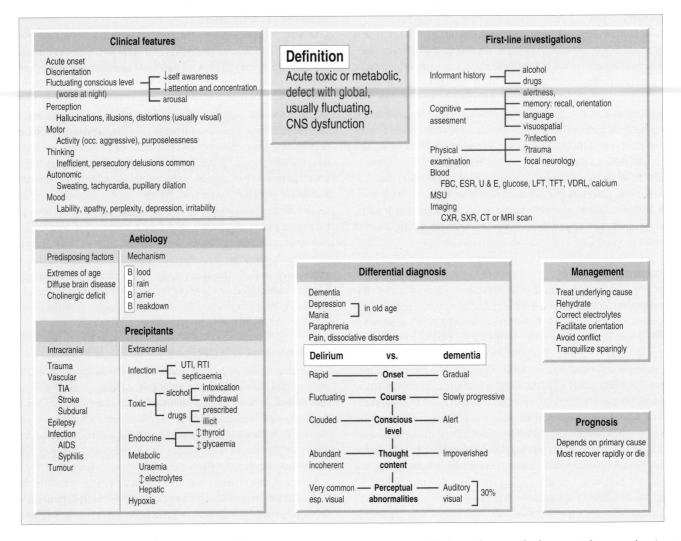

Clinical features

Acute onset
Disorientation
Fluctuating conscious level — ↓self awareness
(worse at night) — ↓attention and concentration
— arousal
Perception
Hallucinations, illusions, distortions (usually visual)
Motor
Activity (occ. aggressive), purposelessness
Thinking
Inefficient, persecutory delusions common
Autonomic
Sweating, tachycardia, pupillary dilation
Mood
Lability, apathy, perplexity, depression, irritability

Definition
Acute toxic or metabolic, defect with global, usually fluctuating, CNS dysfunction

First-line investigations

Informant history — alcohol
— drugs
Cognitive — alertness,
assesment — memory: recall, orientation
— language
— visuospatial
Physical — ?infection
examination — ?trauma
— focal neurology
Blood
FBC, ESR, U & E, glucose, LFT, TFT, VDRL, calcium
MSU
Imaging
CXR, SXR, CT or MRI scan

Aetiology

Predisposing factors	Mechanism
Extremes of age	**B** lood
Diffuse brain disease	**B** rain
Cholinergic deficit	**B** arrier
	B reakdown

Precipitants

Intracranial	Extracranial
Trauma	Infection — UTI, RTI
Vascular	— septicaemia
TIA	Toxic — alcohol — intoxication
Stroke	— withdrawal
Subdural	drugs — prescribed
Epilepsy	— illicit
Infection	Endocrine — ↕thyroid
AIDS	— ↕glycaemia
Syphilis	Metabolic
Tumour	Uraemia
	↕electrolytes
	Hepatic
	Hypoxia

Differential diagnosis

Dementia
Depression — in old age
Mania
Paraphrenia
Pain, dissociative disorders

Delirium	vs.	dementia
Rapid	**Onset**	Gradual
Fluctuating	**Course**	Slowly progressive
Clouded	**Conscious level**	Alert
Abundant incoherent	**Thought content**	Impoverished
Very common esp. visual	**Perceptual abnormalities**	Auditory visual } 30%

Management

Treat underlying cause
Rehydrate
Correct electrolytes
Facilitate orientation
Avoid conflict
Tranquillize sparingly

Prognosis

Depends on primary cause
Most recover rapidly or die

The acute confusional state (also known as delirium) is characterized by the rapid onset of a global but fluctuating dysfunction of the central nervous system (CNS), with an underlying toxic, vascular, ictal or metabolic defect. It represents one of the most important problems encountered in general hospital psychiatry and is seen by a wide range of specialities including general and emergency medicine, general and orthopaedic surgery and medicine for the elderly. It may occur in as many as one-third of older patients admitted to hospital either at initial presentation or during hospitalization.

Clinical features

The most characteristic (although not inevitable) features are an acute onset of *disorientation* and *fluctuating level of consciousness* often worse at night (sundowning). The latter may involve loss of self-awareness, attention and concentration; level of arousal may be heightened or decreased. *Motor activity* may be increased but is usually purposeless; aggressive behaviour occurs in about 10% of cases. *Mood* and affect may fluctuate rapidly (lability) and be accompanied by irritability and/or subjective perplexity; more persistent apathy or depression is also found. *Perceptual disturbances*

are common. Illusions (incorrectly interpreted perceptions) are very common and often frightening; true hallucinations are also common, most frequently visual and usually simple (e.g. geometric patterns or ill-defined shapes). Real objects may appear distorted with size apparently increased or decreased (macro/micropsia). *Thinking* is inefficient; patients complain of being slow and muddled; speech is sometimes incoherent. Poorly systematized, transient delusions are common; these may be secondary to abnormal perceptions and are often persecutory with associated ideas of reference. Sweating, tachycardia and dilated pupils reflect underlying autonomic overactivity. Presentations can be subtle with patients behaving in an uncharacteristic (e.g. withdrawn, saying little) or bizarre fashion (e.g. demanding hospital discharge in the middle of the night): underlying disorientation and impaired consciousness may only become apparent on specific inquiry.

Aetiology
Predisposing factors
Delirium is commonest in the very young and the very old. Those with diffuse brain disease (such as dementia or Parkinson's disease)

are particularly vulnerable, as are those with deficits in cholinergic neurotransmission or taking drugs with anticholinergic properties (e.g. tricyclic antidepressants, procyclidine). Breakdown of the blood–brain barrier is thought to be fundamental. *Precipitants* may be classified as **intracranial** and **extracranial**. Among the former are trauma (e.g. boxing injury) and vascular insults including stroke and haemorrhage (particularly in the subdural space where the presentation may be subacute, and extradurally where sudden collapse may occur after a 'lucid interval'). Epilepsy and intracranial tumour may also present with acute confusion, as may intracranial infection (meningitis, encephalitis or abscess). The great cerebral masqueraders (tuberculosis [TB], neurosyphilis, acquired immunodeficiency syndrome [AIDS]) must always be considered. A wide range of extracranial pathology can result in delirium. Infective causes include urinary tract infection (UTI), pneumonia (which may be 'silent' in old age) and septicaemia. Toxic reactions to drugs frequently cause confusion. Prescribed drugs (including antidepressants, tranquillizers and diuretics) may accumulate in the elderly. Alcohol may confuse both through intoxication (tolerance often decreasing with age) and, most importantly, through withdrawal (delirium tremens [the DTs]). Delirium tremens may occur following abrupt alcohol withdrawal in the context of elective or emergency hospitalization, emphasizing the importance of an accurate alcohol history. Endocrine and metabolic causes of delirium include thyroid hyper- and hypofunction, hyper- and hypoglycaemia (the latter usually more dramatic in onset) and failure of major body systems (heart, lungs, liver, kidneys). Hypoxia is a frequent final common pathway. Nutritional causes (vitamin B_1, B_{12} or folate deficiency) are uncommon, except when secondary to alcohol abuse. In this context, acute vitamin B_1 deficiency (Wernicke's encephalopathy, characterized by ataxia, ophthalmoplegia, nystagmus and confusion) represents a medical emergency since, if untreated, death or irreversible brain damage (Korsakoff's psychosis characterized by short-term memory loss and confabulation) occurs.

Differential diagnosis

Conditions resembling delirium include chronic confusional states (dementias), functional psychiatric conditions (in the elderly, mania and depression as well as paraphrenia should be considered) and responses to major stress, particularly severe pain and dissociative disorders. The diagnosis depends on the demonstration of the cardinal features of delirium (particularly fluctuation in both conscious level and cognitive impairment), the presence of a specific underlying cause and the lack of *consistent* features of affective or psychotic disorders. The differentiation between delirium and dementia may be difficult, since people with established dementia are particularly vulnerable to delirium. Delirium should be considered where deterioration has been rapid, the course is fluctuating (rather than slowly progressive), consciousness is clouded rather than alert, and thought content (which in dementia is usually impoverished) is vivid, complex and muddled. Hallucinations occur both in delirium and dementia. In delirium they are very common and predominantly visual; in dementia, on the other hand, they are as frequently auditory and are only found in about one-third of cases.

Investigations

It is imperative to obtain an informant history, focusing particularly on premorbid level of functioning, onset and course of the confusion and use/abuse of drugs or alcohol. In the mental state assessment, particular attention should be paid to cognitive function (alertness, memory, language, visuospatial ability) and to fluctuation in behaviour. Physical examination is crucial in identifying focal neurological signs and/or evidence of infection or trauma. Essential blood tests include full blood count (FBC) (to exclude anaemia, macrocytosis, leucocytosis), erythrocyte sedimentation rate (ESR) (infection), urea and electrolytes (U & E) (dehydration, electrolyte imbalance), glucose, thyroid and liver function tests (TFT, LFT), calcium and VDRL. Mid-stream urine (MSU) is mandatory and chest and skull X-rays (CXR, SXR) may be informative. Structural brain imaging (computed tomography [CT] or magnetic resonance imaging [MRI]) and electroencephalography (EEG), where available, can identify many intracranial causes.

Management

A high index of suspicion is essential with patients presenting with an acute onset of altered mental functioning and/or disturbed behaviour. Specific management should be targeted at detection of the confusional state itself, and at identification and subsequent treatment of underlying pathology. Patients should therefore usually be managed on general hospital (i.e. not psychiatric) wards. General management includes facilitation of orientation. Patients should be nursed in a quiet well-lit room, avoiding frequent changes in staff. Patients may be very anxious and require consistent explanation and reassurance. Dehydration and electrolyte imbalance are common irrespective of underlying cause and must be corrected. Aggressive outbursts may be minimized by reassurance and the anticipation and avoidance of potential conflict. Where undesirable behaviour must be controlled, antipsychotics are preferable to physical restraint but should be used sparingly; hypotensive and anticholinergic side-effects may precipitate falls or exacerbate the confusion. Haloperidol remains the drug of choice, except when the patient is withdrawing from alcohol or drug abuse, where diazepam is more suitable.

Prognosis

Mortality is high, although dependent on the underlying cause and reduced by rapid diagnosis, identification of any underlying pathology and appropriate general and specific treatment. Where recovery occurs it is usually rapid, with return to premorbid functional level.

18 The dementias

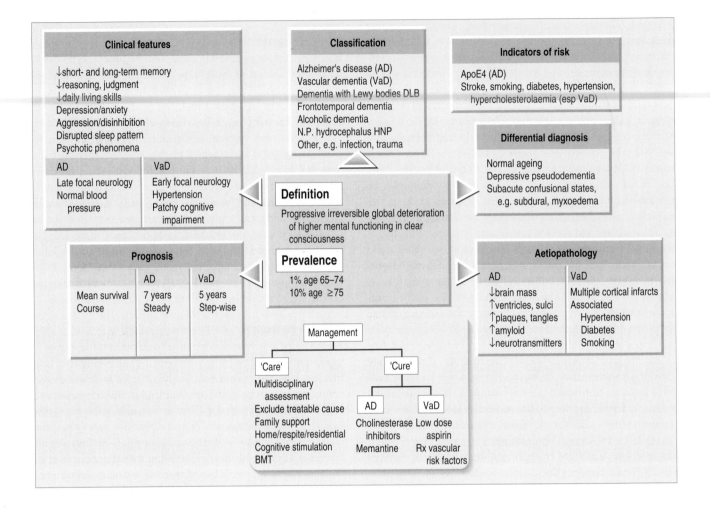

Clinical features

- ↓short- and long-term memory
- ↓reasoning, judgment
- ↓daily living skills
- Depression/anxiety
- Aggression/disinhibition
- Disrupted sleep pattern
- Psychotic phenomena

AD	VaD
Late focal neurology	Early focal neurology
Normal blood pressure	Hypertension
	Patchy cognitive impairment

Classification

Alzheimer's disease (AD)
Vascular dementia (VaD)
Dementia with Lewy bodies DLB
Frontotemporal dementia
Alcoholic dementia
N.P. hydrocephalus HNP
Other, e.g. infection, trauma

Indicators of risk

ApoE4 (AD)
Stroke, smoking, diabetes, hypertension, hypercholesterolaemia (esp VaD)

Differential diagnosis

Normal ageing
Depressive pseudodementia
Subacute confusional states, e.g. subdural, myxoedema

Definition

Progressive irreversible global deterioration of higher mental functioning in clear consciousness

Prevalence

1% age 65–74
10% age ≥75

Prognosis

	AD	VaD
Mean survival	7 years	5 years
Course	Steady	Step-wise

Aetiopathology

AD	VaD
↓brain mass	Multiple cortical infarcts
↑ventricles, sulci	Associated
↑plaques, tangles	Hypertension
↑amyloid	Diabetes
↓neurotransmitters	Smoking

Management

'Care'
- Multidisciplinary assessment
- Exclude treatable cause
- Family support
- Home/respite/residential
- Cognitive stimulation
- BMT

'Cure'

AD	VaD
Cholinesterase inhibitors	Low dose aspirin
Memantine	Rx vascular risk factors

Definition and clinical presentation

Dementia is a syndrome rather than a diagnosis, referring to a progressive and (usually) irreversible global deterioration of higher mental functioning in clear consciousness. The most obvious manifestations are disruption of memory (long- and short-term), language (nominal aphasia being particularly common) and 'intelligence' in terms of reasoning, judgment and performance in IQ tests. Other features include changes in personality and behaviour, reflected both in loss of daily living skills (e.g. washing, dressing, handling money) and in abnormal behaviours, including aggression, wandering and sexual disinhibition. Apathy, depression and anxiety are frequent and there may be disturbances of sleep, including daytime drowsiness, confusion between day and night and nocturnal restlessness. Psychotic phenomena, particularly persecutory delusions (aggravated by forgetfulness) and auditory or visual hallucinations occur in one-third of patients. Dementia interferes with the sufferer's family, work and social functioning. Presentation seldom occurs until the dementia has been present for at least 1 year and is often at family instigation. The clinical presentation may differ between types of dementia.

Epidemiology

Dementia becomes commoner with increasing age. Onset before the age of 65 years is rare. One per cent of the population aged 65–74 years, 10% of those aged 75+ years and 25% of those aged 85+ years are affected. As the 'very old' population in the developed world increases, the absolute number of those with dementia will rise more steeply, as will the burden of providing adequate dementia care.

Classification

The major dementias are degenerative. These include Alzheimer's disease (AD, about 50% of cases) and the vascular dementias (VaD—20–30% of cases) VaD is associated with more patchy cognitive impairment than AD, focal neurological symptoms or signs and a 'stepwise' rather than continuous deterioration. It is increasingly recognized that a high proportion of people with dementia have a mixed picture and that patterns of progression differ less than previously thought between AD and VaD. Dementia with Lewy bodies (DLB), characterized by fluctuating cognitive functioning, visual hallucinations, sensitivity to neuroleptic side-effects and parkinsonian features may account for as many as 20% of people with dementia. Frontotemporal dementia has a younger mean age of onset and accounts for up to 20% of early-onset dementias, and is characterized by early personality changes and relative intellectual sparing. Dementia in the context of chronic alcohol abuse accounts for up to 10% of cases. More rarely, dementia may be associated with repeated head trauma (as in boxers), subdural haematoma, Huntington's chorea or infection (human immunodeficiency virus [HIV], syphilis, prion). Normal pressure hydrocephalus (NPH) may be idiopathic or due to subarachnoid haemorrhage, head injury or meningitis. NPH produces a 'patchy' dementia with marked mental slowness, apathy and early onset of gait abnormalities and loss of control of micturition. Ventriculoatrial shunting may benefit up to 50% of cases.

Aetiopathology

1 AD. At macroscopic level (and on computed tomography [CT] or magnetic resonance imaging [MRI] scan), the brain in AD is shrunken, with increased sulcal widening and enlarged ventricles. Microscopically, the key changes are neuronal loss and the presence (particularly in cortex and hippocampus) of 'amyloid plaques' (containing a core of amyloid protein) and neurofibrillary tangles. Neurochemically, there are deficits in several neurotransmitters including acetylcholine, noradrenaline, serotonin and somatostatin, with corresponding loss of the cell bodies of neurones secreting these transmitters. Hypotheses relating to free radical damage and amyloid toxicity have been proposed to explain why neurones degenerate in AD. Studies of rare familial forms of early-onset AD, where inheritance is autosomal dominant, have led to the discovery of a number of specific abnormalities in genes coding for the amyloid precursor protein (APP), which increase production of β-A4 peptide fragments of APP forming the core of amyloid plaques. Inheritance of late-onset AD is complex, polygenic and multifactorial. The apolipoprotein E (ApoE) gene may be a clinically useful marker of risk in subjects with late-onset, non-familial AD. Three common alleles (E2, E3, E4) exist; the E4 allele (particularly if homozygous) appears to indicate increased risk and earlier onset. Low childhood educational attainment and mental inactivity also increase the risk of late-life dementia.

2 VaD is associated with multiple areas of cortical infarction. Damage to deep white matter vasculature may also cause dementia. There is a ninefold increase in risk of dementia in the year after a stroke, and vascular risk factors such as hypertension, hypercholesterolaemia, diabetes and smoking are also risk factors for dementia. These may also be risk factors for AD.

3 DLB is associated with the presence in the cerebral cortex of Lewy bodies identical to those found in the basal ganglia in Parkinson's disease. Pathological changes characteristic of AD are also often found.

4 Frontotemporal dementias mainly affect the frontal and anterior temporal lobes; about 25% exhibit Pick-type histological changes.

Differential diagnosis

Many normal elderly people develop mild, circumscribed deterioration in memory. They may need reassurance that they do not have a dementia. Severe depression in old age may present with a 'pseudodementia' with prominent forgetfulness and poor self-care. Such patients usually have a short history and are often aware of, and distressed by, their poor function. Slowly progressive acute confusional states (e.g. subdural haematoma, myxoedema and vitamin deficiencies) may present with a dementia-like picture.

Management

There may be some functional improvement in patients with VaD in whom vascular risk factors for stroke are controlled; low-dose aspirin also reduces risk of further stroke-related deterioration. Cholinesterase inhibitors (donepezil, rivastigmine, galantamine) are currently recommended for symptomatic treatment of cognitive and behavioural deficits in mild to moderate AD. Usefulness in other forms of dementia is being investigated. Memantine, which modulates glutamate neurotransmission, is licensed for the treatment of moderate to severe AD. Patients should have a full multidisciplinary assessment to exclude treatable causes and identify specific problems. The possibility of superadded and treatable acute confusional states (commonly iatrogenic or secondary to infection) should always be considered if a patient deteriorates. Depression often complicates established dementia and may respond to antidepressants.

The focus of management of dementia must be on care delivery, assessing and responding to the changing needs of affected patients and their family carers, and maintaining dignity and individuality. Support may include home-care input as well as day and intermittent respite in social service or hospital settings. Patients with severe dementia may require residential, nursing or hospital care. Psychological techniques such as cognitive stimulation or behavioural management techniques (BMT) may improve cognition and behaviour.

Prognosis

Patients with AD usually deteriorate inexorably to an endstage needing full nursing care; death is often from bronchopneumonia, though very elderly patients frequently die of other causes before the dementia becomes severe. VaD has a slightly worse prognosis; progression is less consistent with vulnerability to sudden stroke-related death. Skilled nursing care may substantially increase life expectancy in very severe dementia.

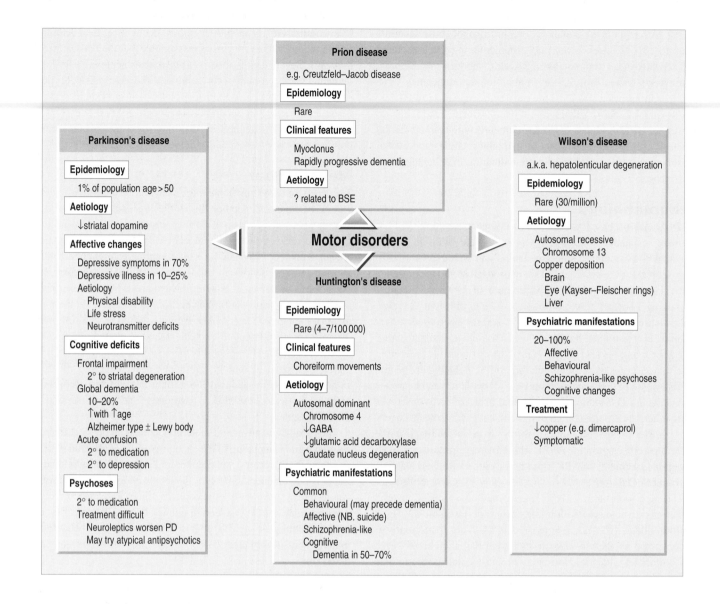

Prion disease

e.g. Creutzfeld–Jacob disease

Epidemiology

Rare

Clinical features

Myoclonus
Rapidly progressive dementia

Aetiology

? related to BSE

Parkinson's disease

Epidemiology

1% of population age > 50

Aetiology

↓striatal dopamine

Affective changes

Depressive symptoms in 70%
Depressive illness in 10–25%
Aetiology
    Physical disability
    Life stress
    Neurotransmitter deficits

Cognitive deficits

Frontal impairment
    2° to striatal degeneration
Global dementia
    10–20%
    ↑with ↑age
    Alzheimer type ± Lewy body
Acute confusion
    2° to medication
    2° to depression

Psychoses

2° to medication
Treatment difficult
    Neuroleptics worsen PD
    May try atypical antipsychotics

Motor disorders

Huntington's disease

Epidemiology

Rare (4–7/100 000)

Clinical features

Choreiform movements

Aetiology

Autosomal dominant
    Chromosome 4
    ↓GABA
    ↓glutamic acid decarboxylase
    Caudate nucleus degeneration

Psychiatric manifestations

Common
    Behavioural (may precede dementia)
    Affective (NB. suicide)
    Schizophrenia-like
    Cognitive
        Dementia in 50–70%

Wilson's disease

a.k.a. hepatolenticular degeneration

Epidemiology

Rare (30/million)

Aetiology

Autosomal recessive
    Chromosome 13
Copper deposition
    Brain
    Eye (Kayser–Fleischer rings)
    Liver

Psychiatric manifestations

20–100%
    Affective
    Behavioural
    Schizophrenia-like psychoses
    Cognitive changes

Treatment

↓copper (e.g. dimercaprol)
Symptomatic

Neuropsychiatry is primarily concerned with those conditions in which mental disorder results from demonstrable structural or neurophysiological disturbance of the brain. There are several ways of classifying these disorders, including focal and diffuse, specific and global and according to aetiology. Cerebral causes include degenerative (dementias, Parkinson's disease, Huntington's disease), infections (syphilis, acquired immunodeficiency syndrome [AIDS]), epilepsy and miscellaneous (multiple sclerosis, Wilson's disease). Systemic causes include metabolic disturbances (e.g. porphyria), endocrinopathies and vitamin deficiencies.

In general, the psychiatric aspects of organic disorders may be divided into personality and behavioural changes, cognitive difficulties, affective disturbances, psychoses and drug-induced problems, for example confusional states. The psychiatric picture seldom bears a specific relationship to the type of underlying pathology, being more influenced by the site of brain involvement and the time course of the illness. The presentation is also coloured by the patient's premorbid personality, predisposition to psychiatric disorder and social circumstances. An organic disorder can mimic functional disorders, but points in favour of organic problems, including cognitive disorder preceding mood or other disorder, specific cognitive deficits, neurological signs, fluctuating symptomatology, visual hallucinations, vague or transient paranoid delusions and symptoms not typical of a functional disorder. In order to make the diagnosis, a full psychiatric history and mental state examination (see Chapter 1), and full physical and neurological examinations must be undertaken. Special investigations should include a general screen (see Chapter 17). Where a specific diagnosis is suspected, more specific investigations (as detailed under individual conditions below) may help in its confirmation. Lumbar puncture should be undertaken with caution if raised intracranial pressure is suspected in view of the risk of precipitating brainstem coning.

Dementias are sometimes classified as cortical or subcortical, although neither type exclusively affects only cortical or subcortical tissue. Subcortical dementias include Parkinson's disease, Huntington's disease and progressive supra-nuclear palsy. Symptoms include psychomotor slowing and executive dysfunction associated with disruption to frontal pathways, in addition to disease-specific symptoms. Subcortical dementias are rarely associated with focal cognitive symptoms such as aphasia or agnosia.

Parkinson's disease (PD)

PD, affecting over 1% of the population above 50 years of age, results from deficient striatal dopaminergic activity. Psychiatric disturbances are common and include intellectual impairment, affective changes and psychoses. Global dementia occurs in 10–20% of PD patients over 65 years (associated mainly with the neuropathological changes of Alzheimer's disease and dementia with Lewy bodies), with increasing age being an important contributory factor. Frontal lobe cognitive deficits are seen early in PD and relate to striatal dysfunction. Isolated focal abnormalities (e.g. immediate recall of verbal material, working memory), drug-induced confusional states (especially with antimuscarinic compounds and selegiline) and depression-related cognitive difficulties are also common. Thirty per cent of PD patients develop psychotic phenomena, probably in relation to their anti-PD medication. Affective disturbances (depressive symptoms [70%], depressive illness [10–25%]) may be confounded by physical symptoms of PD and are complex in aetiology, with both neurotransmitter systems (dopaminergic, serotonergic, cholinergic) and social problems (low self-esteem, physical disability, poorly targeted coping strategies, dissatisfaction with support, social stress, sexual problems) being invoked. The degree of motor disability does not correlate strongly with abnormalities of mood, although depression may be encountered more often in patients with prominent gait and postural changes. Treatment of depression and psychoses should, where possible, be with drugs less liable to induce neurological side-effects to which such patients are particularly vulnerable. Atypical antipsychotics may be useful, although extreme caution is required in the context of dementia (see Chapter 33).

Huntington's disease (HD)

HD, characterized by cognitive decline, choreiform involuntary movements and 'fidgetiness', is inherited as an autosomal dominant gene (100% penetrance) on the short arm of chromosome 4. Rare individuals have a negative family history, which may be due to a new spontaneous mutation or illegitimacy. HD manifests at 25–50 years of age, affects men and women equally, and prevalence is 4–7/100 000. There is cerebral atrophy, and reduced γ-aminobutyric acid (GABA) resulting in dopamine hypersensitivity (especially

caudate and putamen). Psychiatric disturbances, common in both individuals at risk and in patients with HD, include changes in behaviour/personality (apathy, irritability), affective disorders (depression = 40%; mania = 10%) and schizophreniform psychoses as well as cognitive impairment or frank dementia (50–70% of patients with chorea). The dementia is subcortical, characterized by poor cognitive function, mental slowing and a decline in memory, but no dysfunction of language and no focal deficits of perception. Many patients with HD have insight into their intellectual impairment (which may precede other symptoms). Depression can also precede other symptoms and occurs in a subset of families. There is an increased risk of suicide both in patients with HD and in those at risk, and this must be borne in mind when planning genetic counselling and predictive testing. Treatment for HD is symptomatic, and depression and psychoses should be treated with standard medications. Death occurs about 15 years after diagnosis.

Hepatolenticular degeneration

Hepatolenticular degeneration, also known as Wilson's disease (WD), is an uncommon inborn error of metabolism (estimated at 30/million) transmitted by an autosomal recessive gene (mapped to chromosome 13) and characterized by an accumulation of copper in the liver, brain, kidney, cornea (Kayser–Fleischer rings) and bone. WD is characterized by abnormal movements (e.g. generalized tremor, dystonia), muscular rigidity, dysarthria, dysphagia and cirrhosis of the liver. Psychiatric manifestations occur in 20–100% and may be the presenting feature. The most common psychiatric symptom clusters are affective (e.g. emotional lability, irritability, incongruity, anxiety, depression, mania) and behavioural changes (e.g. aggressive, antisocial). Schizophrenia-like psychoses are uncommon. Cognitive changes are well recognized (deficits in memory, visuospatial and learning skills, learning disability, dementia) and occur in those with neurological rather than hepatic impairment and with abnormalities of the basal ganglia on computed tomography (CT) scan. Treatment is with 'anticopper drugs' (e.g. dimercaprol, penicillamine, trientine); psychiatric disturbances are treated with antidepressants or antipsychotics.

Prion disease

Human forms of *spongiform encephalopathy* (prion disorders, e.g. Creutzfeld–Jacob disease [CJD]) are characterized by accumulation of an abnormal form of a normal host protease-resistant protein (PrP) in the brain. They present with a rapidly fatal dementia associated with myoclonic jerks. CJD is familial (15%; sometimes autosomal dominant) and the incidence is 1/million per year. These disorders also occur in animals, for example bovine spongiform encephalopathy (BSE—'mad cow disease') and scrapie. A link has been established between BSE and 'new form', early-onset, human CJD.

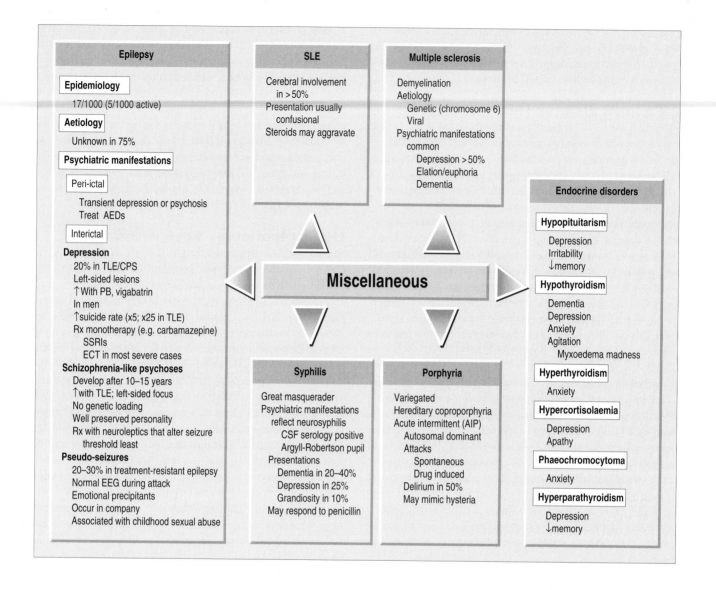

Epilepsy

Epidemiology
17/1000 (5/1000 active)

Aetiology
Unknown in 75%

Psychiatric manifestations

Peri-ictal
Transient depression or psychosis
Treat AEDs

Interictal

Depression
20% in TLE/CPS
Left-sided lesions
↑With PB, vigabatrin
In men
↑suicide rate (x5; x25 in TLE)
Rx monotherapy (e.g. carbamazepine)
SSRIs
ECT in most severe cases
Schizophrenia-like psychoses
Develop after 10–15 years
↑with TLE; left-sided focus
No genetic loading
Well preserved personality
Rx with neuroleptics that alter seizure threshold least
Pseudo-seizures
20–30% in treatment-resistant epilepsy
Normal EEG during attack
Emotional precipitants
Occur in company
Associated with childhood sexual abuse

SLE
Cerebral involvement in >50%
Presentation usually confusional
Steroids may aggravate

Multiple sclerosis
Demyelination
Aetiology
Genetic (chromosome 6)
Viral
Psychiatric manifestations common
Depression >50%
Elation/euphoria
Dementia

Miscellaneous

Syphilis
Great masquerader
Psychiatric manifestations reflect neurosyphilis
CSF serology positive
Argyll-Robertson pupil
Presentations
Dementia in 20–40%
Depression in 25%
Grandiosity in 10%
May respond to penicillin

Porphyria
Variegated
Hereditary coproporphyria
Acute intermittent (AIP)
Autosomal dominant
Attacks
Spontaneous
Drug induced
Delirium in 50%
May mimic hysteria

Endocrine disorders

Hypopituitarism
Depression
Irritability
↓memory

Hypothyroidism
Dementia
Depression
Anxiety
Agitation
Myxoedema madness

Hyperthyroidism
Anxiety

Hypercortisolaemia
Depression
Apathy

Phaeochromocytoma
Anxiety

Hyperparathyroidism
Depression
↓memory

Epilepsy

Epilepsy is common (lifetime prevalence = 17/1000; prevalence of active epilepsy = 5/1000), affecting men more. Age at onset is usually before 30 years (75%), the commonest seizure type being complex partial (60%), 90% arising in temporal lobes. Aetiology is unknown in the majority of cases (75%). Psychiatric aspects of epilepsy may be divided into peri-ictal (relating to the ictus or seizures) and interictal (disturbances are chronic and not related to the ictal electric discharge). Depression is common in people with epilepsy (PWE), the commonest and clinically relevant entity being interictal depression. Mania and elation are rare. Depression, which may be severe and rapid in onset, is more likely to occur in patients with temporal lobe epilepsy (TLE)/complex partial seizures (CPS), of whom 20% become depressed. There may be a decrease in seizure frequency prior to the depression and a predominance of left-sided lesions. Other neuroepilepsy variables (e.g. age of onset

of epilepsy, presence of an intracranial lesion) do not seem related to depression. Aetiological factors include antiepileptic drugs (AEDs) (e.g. phenobarbitone [PB] and vigabatrin), genetic predisposition, gender (possibly men more) and psychosocial factors (adverse life events, poor adjustment to seizures, social stigmatization, financial stress, unemployment). Suicide is increased in PWE (5 × general population; TLE 25 ×). Treatment includes AED monotherapy (e.g. carbamazepine [improves mood] if possible), careful use of antidepressants as most (except monoamine oxidase inhibitors [MAOIs]) lower the seizure threshold (selective serotonin reuptake inhibitors [SSRIs] possibly better) and electroconvulsive therapy (ECT) if necessary. There is an increased incidence of 'interictal' schizophrenia-like psychoses (usually paranoid) in PWE. The psychoses (which usually develop 10–15 years after onset of epilepsy) are associated with left TLE, neurological abnormalities, negative family history of schizophrenia and a 'warm' affect with little personality deterioration. Treatment is with antipsychotics which lower the seizure threshold relatively little (e.g. haloperidol). Cognitive changes are common in PWE and may be caused by AEDs (PB, phenytoin) or persistent abnormal electrical activity in the brain between seizures. Pseudo-seizures simulate real seizures and occur in 20–30% of people with chronic treatment-resistant epilepsy. They are often frequent, occur when others are present, indoors or at home, have an emotional precipitant and are associated with a history of childhood sexual abuse. Characteristically, the electroencephalography (EEG) (during the attack) and the serum prolactin (after the attack) are normal. Most PWE have a normal personality and when a personality disorder does occur it is not of any particular kind. Sexual dysfunction is common in PWE (causes include the effect of AEDs, neurophysiological problems [more common in TLE] and social problems).

Multiple sclerosis (MS)

MS is common and characterized by episodes of demyelination which result in central nervous system (CNS) abnormalities disseminated in time and space. Both genetics (chromosome 6 possibly responsible) and environment (e.g. virus) are aetiologically important. Psychiatric manifestations include personality changes, elation/euphoria (often associated with cognitive impairment), depression (>50%), suicide, cognitive impairment (early on) and progressive dementia (late stages). Denial of disability is common.

Syphilis

Syphilis (*Treponema pallidum* infection) has three stages: primary (chancre at the site of inoculation), secondary (cutaneous rashes, condylomata, mucous patches, lymphadenopathy) and tertiary (rare today but including meningovascular and parenchymatous [optic atrophy, general paralysis of the insane (GPI), tabes dorsalis] subtypes). Positive cerebrospinal fluid (CSF) serology and raised CSF protein (neurosyphilis) occurs in the tertiary stage, may be asymptomatic or can present with any type of psychiatric symptomatology. Meningovascular syphilis appears 1–5 years after the primary infection and can present with headache, malaise, lethargy, irritability, delirium or dementia. Tabes dorsalis, appearing 8–12 years after the primary infection, presents with lightning pains, ataxia, paraesthesias and Argyll-Robertson pupils (small, irregular, reactive to convergence but not to light). GPI, appearing 5–25 years after the primary infection, has an insidious onset. There may be personality (disinhibition, irritability, lability) and cognitive (poor concentration) changes, dementia (20–40%), depression (25%), grandiosity (10%) and, more rarely, mania and schizophrenia-like psychoses. Intramuscular penicillin remains the first-line treatment and may induce neuropsychiatric improvement even in advanced disease.

Porphyria

Porphyria consists of three types: acute intermittent porphyria (AIP), hereditary coproporphyria and variegate porphyria; all are rare. AIP is a metabolic error of haem breakdown which leads to porphobilinogen in urine, is transmitted by an autosomal dominant gene with variable penetrance and is slightly more common in women (female/male = 3 : 2). AIP is characterized by acute attacks which may occur spontaneously or may be precipitated by drugs (barbiturates, sulphonamides, methyldopa, oral contraception, hypoglycaemics, alcohol), infections, pregnancy, metabolic and nutritional factors (e.g. low carbohydrate intake). Clinical presentation may be abdominal (colicky pain, vomiting, constipation) and neurological (peripheral neuropathy, bulbar palsies, epilepsy). Psychiatric disturbances are found more often in AIP than in any other form of porphyria and include delirium (50%), depression, emotional lability, schizophrenia-like psychoses (especially paranoid) and symptoms incorrectly diagnosed as 'hysteria'. It has been claimed that the psychiatric disorders of King George III were manifestations of porphyria.

Systemic lupus erythematosus (SLE)

SLE is a connective tissue disorder which can present with skin changes, renal involvement, arthritis and cerebral SLE (>50%). Characteristically, there are transient, fluctuating psychiatric disturbances of which the acute organic reaction is commonest. Depressive psychosis may occur less frequently. Transient psychotic phenomena may occur although persistent schizophrenia-like psychoses are rare. Treatment with steroids may cause further psychiatric complications.

Endocrine

Endocrine causes of psychiatric symptoms include pituitary, thyroid, adrenal and parathyroid abnormalities. Hypopituitarism (Simmond's disease) is almost invariably associated with depression, irritability and/or impaired memory. Hypothyroidism may present as dementia, depression, anxiety or acute agitation (myxoedema madness—with features of predominantly agitated depression). Hyperthyroidism can be associated with anxiety or depression (which may be delusional). Hypercortisolaemia, which is most commonly iatrogenic, may induce depression or mania. Hypocortisolaemia (Addison's disease) is usually associated with depression and apathy. Phaeochromocytoma may present with episodic anxiety accompanied by labile hypertension. Hyperparathyroidism is often accompanied by depression and apathy and occasionally by memory deficits.

Vitamin B$_{12}$

Vitamin B$_{12}$ deficiency results in pernicious anaemia and may be accompanied by subacute combined degeneration of the spinal cord associated with signs of neuropathy and spinal cord involvement. Psychiatric symptoms include slowing of mental processes, confusion, memory problems, intellectual impairment (all associated with low serum B$_{12}$), depression and paranoid delusions. Treatment is with hydroxycobalamin.

School absence

	Refusal	Truancy
Whereabouts	Known	Not known
Associated psychopathology	Anxiety	Conduct disorder
Academic performance	Good	Poor
Family history	Anxiety, depression	Antisocial personality
Family type	Small	Large, deprived

Child abuse

Types

Physical
- Child battering (NAI)
- Psychosocial dwarfism
- Munchausen by proxy

Emotional

Sexual

Vulnerability factors

Child
- Unwanted
- Low birth weight
- Handicap (mental/physical)
- Early separation from mother
- Persistent restlessness/crying

Parent
- Young and/or single
- History of abuse
- Unemployment
- Poverty

Signs
- Unexplained injuries
- Fear of parents
- Failure to thrive

Consequences
- Emotional, conduct and developmental discorders
- Depression
- Conversion disorders
- Child-rearing problems

Management
- Detection
- Confrontation
- Protection
- Individual/family therapy

Conduct disorders

Prevalence

4%
↑in males
↑in low social class

Clinical features

Antisocial
Delinquency

Types

Socialized (peer acceptance)
Unsocialized (peer rejection)

Aetiology

Harsh/violent parenting
Eductional failure
ADHD
Learning/communication disorders
Family
  Disharmony
  Psychiatric illness

Prognosis

Better if 'socialized'
2/3 persist in adulthood

Psychotic disorders

Rare

Types

Schizophrenia
Disintegrative psychoses

Emotional disorders

Anxiety

Commonest emotional disorder in childhood
Autonomic, psychological and somatic components
Phobias usually not clinically significant

Depression

Prevalence 1%
Phenomenology ≃ adult
Suicide rare (M=F)
Parasuicide common (F>M)
Treatment, psychological therapies

Psychiatric assessment of children

The assessment will involve interview(s) with the child and with informants (usually parents and a teacher). The informant history must cover the presenting problem (nature, precipitants, alleviators, effect on family), other current behavioural or emotional difficulties (including mood, sleep, appetite, elimination, relationships and antisocial behaviours), school behaviour and academic performance, daily routine (including hobbies), personal history (pregnancy, milestones, past illnesses/injuries/hospitalizations, abuse, etc.) and family structure and function (parental characteristics, quality of parenting, family interactions, past or current separations). Direct assessment of the child's behaviour will focus on his/her appearance (including signs of neglect or injury), nature and level of spontaneous activity, affect, rapport with interviewer, interaction with parent(s), mannerisms and psychotic features. Physical examination, including neurological screening, is an important element of the initial assessment.

Classification

The classification of child psychiatric disorders is broadly divided into conduct disorders and emotional disorders (which may coexist), developmental disorders (global, pervasive or specific), disorders of elimination, hyperkinetic disorders, psychotic disorders, psychiatric aspects of child abuse and disorders of sleep.

Conduct (behavioural) disorders

These are characterized by persistent antisocial behaviours, such as disobedience, lying, truancy, aggression, stealing, promiscuity and damage to property (including fire setting). The prevalence is 4% with a male/female ratio of 3:1 and a marked lower social class preponderance. Low self-esteem and poor peer relationships are present in 20%; these are classified as 'mixed' conduct/emotional disorders. The term 'delinquency' refers to the subgroup who break the law. Conduct disorders may be classified into 'socialized' (where the antisocial behaviours are viewed as normal within the peer group and/or family) and 'unsocialized' where the antisocial behaviour is solitary and associated with peer and parental rejection. Aetiological factors include family disharmony, harsh inconsistent parenting with frequent parental violence, aggression, alcoholism, antisocial personality disorder and depression. Conduct disorder is linked strongly to educational failure, and may coexist with attention-deficit hyperactivity disorder (ADHD), learning and/or communication disorders. Management usually involves a combination of family therapy, behavioural treatment of aggression and remedial teaching as well as the provision of alternative peer group activities. Antisocial behaviours persist into adult life in two-thirds; the prognosis is better in the 'socialized' group.

Emotional disorders

These are present in 2–3% of children with a female preponderance and a generally favourable prognosis. The major subtypes are described below; recent classificatory systems have proposed additional categories including social sensitivity, separation anxiety, hypochondriasis, conversion disorders and sibling rivalry. In general, treatment involves a combination of behavioural and family therapy.

School refusal (or school phobia) accounts for 1% of school absences, with no gender or social class differences and peaks at ages 5 and 11 years. The presentation may be with somatic symptoms (headache, abdominal pain). Three peak ages are recognized: younger children of 5–6 years (separation anxiety); children aged 10–11 years (school transition); and adolescents (low self-esteem which may in turn reflect an underlying depression). Parents (often overprotective with no excess of marital discord) are aware and often collude. Treatment is aimed at graded or abrupt resumption of school attendance. Outcome is good in 60%, although one-third have neurotic disorders in adulthood.

Generalized anxiety, the most common emotional disorder in childhood, has both autonomic (palpitations, dry mouth) and psychological (fear) components. Somatic symptoms, particularly abdominal pain, are also common. Predisposing factors include the child's temperament and parental overprotection.

Phobias, particularly of the dark or of strangers, are common in small children and usually are not clinically significant. When persistent and intense (often in response to parental or social reinforcement) the consequent avoidance may become pathological.

Depression is characterized, as in adults, by pervasive low mood, anhedonia, altered sleep and appetite, depressive cognitions, including reduced self-esteem, and self-destructive thoughts. It is distinguished by severity and persistence from normal sadness and it should be noted that fleeting suicidal thoughts are quite common in healthy pre-adolescents. Recent evidence (using structured clinical interviews) suggests a prevalence for depression of 1% in pre-pubertal children. Treatment may involve psychological therapies and—if depression is moderate to severe with biological features—antidepressants may be tried. There is, however, increasing concern both about limited efficacy and the possibility of precipitating suicidal or aggressive behaviour. Completed suicide is rare in children, equal in boys and girls, and there is no particular class distribution. Attempted suicide is more common, girls attempting three times more than boys, and has a higher incidence in lower socio-economic classes.

Bereavement reactions are common and characterized by prolonged sadness, irritability, guilt and crying, which may last for several months with similar stages of grief to those experienced by adults. Enuresis and temper tantrums may be precipitated in younger children, while in older children sleep disturbance, poor school performance and depressive illness may ensue. The surviving parent's coping mechanisms are crucial.

Obsessive–compulsive disorder (OCD) is rare in early childhood (prevalence 0.3%), although isolated compulsions (not walking on paving stone lines) are common. OCD presents much as in adults and usually responds to a combination of cognitive behavioural methods (usually requiring family cooperation). Fluoxetine may be tried cautiously in this age-group.

Child abuse

The concept covers neglect and emotional abuse as well as sexual and/or physical assault (including non-accidental injury [NAI]). Abuse can occur in all social strata and a high index of suspicion is crucial. Vulnerability factors in the child include being unwanted, having a low birth weight, early maternal separation, mental or physical handicap and persistent restlessness or crying. Young and/or single parents with their own history of abuse, adverse socio-economic circumstances (particularly unemployment) and unrealistic styles of disciplining are particularly liable to abuse their children. Signs of abuse include injuries without convincing explanation, previous history of similar injury and evidence in the child of withdrawal and/or fear of parents. Emotional abuse is an important cause of non-organic 'failure to thrive'. Psychiatric consequences of child abuse include increased vulnerability to subsequent emotional, conduct and developmental disorders later in childhood, as well as depression, conversion disorders (e.g. pseudo-seizures) and child rearing problems in adult life. Management involves detection, confrontation, arranging protection for the child if necessary and individual and family therapy.

Sleep problems

These are common in normal children with restless sleep in 30%, night-time wakefulness in 20% and sleep-talking in 10%. Night terrors, in which children sit up terrified and screaming but cannot be woken sufficiently to be reassured, have a peak incidence (3%) at age 4–7 years and a frequently positive family history. They arise from deep (stage 4) sleep and are accompanied by tachycardia and tachypnoea. They are aggravated by daytime stress and usually resolve spontaneously. Nightmares (peak incidence age 5–6 years) may be equally frightening and are also often stress related; the child can, however, be easily woken and reassured.

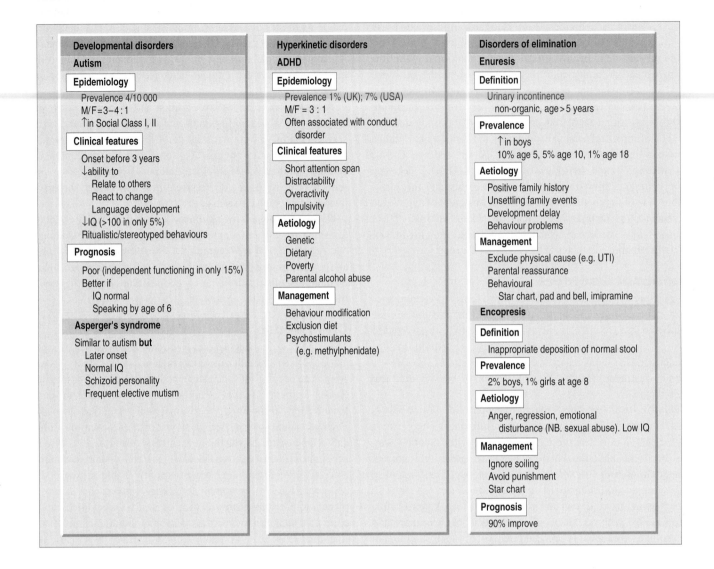

Developmental disorders

Autism

Epidemiology
Prevalence 4/10 000
M/F = 3–4 : 1
↑in Social Class I, II

Clinical features
Onset before 3 years
↓ability to
  Relate to others
  React to change
  Language development
↓IQ (>100 in only 5%)
Ritualistic/stereotyped behaviours

Prognosis
Poor (independent functioning in only 15%)
Better if
  IQ normal
  Speaking by age of 6

Asperger's syndrome
Similar to autism **but**
  Later onset
  Normal IQ
  Schizoid personality
  Frequent elective mutism

Hyperkinetic disorders

ADHD

Epidemiology
Prevalence 1% (UK); 7% (USA)
M/F = 3 : 1
Often associated with conduct
  disorder

Clinical features
Short attention span
Distractability
Overactivity
Impulsivity

Aetiology
Genetic
Dietary
Poverty
Parental alcohol abuse

Management
Behaviour modification
Exclusion diet
Psychostimulants
  (e.g. methylphenidate)

Disorders of elimination

Enuresis

Definition
Urinary incontinence
  non-organic, age > 5 years

Prevalence
↑ in boys
10% age 5, 5% age 10, 1% age 18

Aetiology
Positive family history
Unsettling family events
Development delay
Behaviour problems

Management
Exclude physical cause (e.g. UTI)
Parental reassurance
Behavioural
  Star chart, pad and bell, imipramine

Encopresis

Definition
Inappropriate deposition of normal stool

Prevalence
2% boys, 1% girls at age 8

Aetiology
Anger, regression, emotional
  disturbance (NB. sexual abuse). Low IQ

Management
Ignore soiling
Avoid punishment
Star chart

Prognosis
90% improve

Developmental disorders

Autism is the most important pervasive developmental disorder (PDD). It is present in about 4/10 000 children with a male/female ratio of 3–4 : 1 and is more common in Social Classes I and II. Essential features of the disorders are an inability to relate to other people and to changing situations. The onset is before the age of 36 months and can even occur in the first few months (called 'no onset' type). Three features are regarded as essential to the diagnosis: a pervasive failure to make social relationships (aloofness, lack of eye contact, etc.); major defects in language development; and resistance to change with associated ritualistic and/or manneristic behaviours. These may all reflect an inability to process emotional cues. Psychotic phenomena are absent. Affected children often develop inappropriate attachments to unusual objects, have a restricted range of interests and activities, exhibit stereotyped behaviours (rocking, twirling, etc.) and have unpredictable outbursts of screaming or laughter. Although the majority are of limited intelligence (IQ > 100 in only 5%), some autistic children have isolated skills (rote memory, computation). Learning disability, deafness and childhood schizophrenia must be considered in the differential diagnosis. Organic factors are strongly implicated in the aetiology: these include genetic loading and perinatal complications. Associated genetic disorders include tuberous sclerosis and Fragile X syndrome. Behavioural treatments, particularly operant conditioning, may reduce stereotypies and encourage more normal development and social functioning. Family support and counselling is crucial. Prognosis is poor with persistent impairments in 60% and further deterioration in 20%; only 15% achieve fully independent functioning. Outcome is considerably better in those with a non-verbal IQ over 70 and if speech has developed by the age of 6 years. *Asperger's syndrome* is a less severe form of PDD with later onset, normal intelligence and schizoid personality. Pedantic speech and a preoccupation with obscure facts often occur.

Elective mutism is a marked, emotionally determined selectivity in speaking, such that a child is able to comprehend spoken language, demonstrates language competence in some social situations but fails to speak in others. Milder forms of the disorder are common but short-lived (usually at the beginning of schooling), while a clinically significant form is present in 1/1000. Affected children are usually very shy but stubborn and may have had previous speech delay; parents are often overprotective. Recovery occurs in about 50%; those not improving by the age of 10 years usually do badly.

Specific reading retardation (SRR) represents reading difficulties that interfere with academic progress and is not accounted for by low intelligence, poor schooling or visual or auditory difficulties. Prevalence is between 5% and 10% with a marked male and working-class preponderance. Neuropsychological testing often reveals perceptual and/or language deficits and there may be coexistent attention-deficit hyperactivity disorder (ADHD).

Disorders of elimination

Enuresis refers to non-organic involuntary bladder emptying after the age of 5 years. It can occur by day, by night or both, and is defined as secondary if there has been a period of urinary continence and primary if not. Prevalence is 10% at age 5, 5% at age 10 and 1% at age 18 years. The male/female ratio is 2:1. Aetiological factors include positive family history, unsettling family events, developmental delay and other behavioural problems in the child. Management involves the exclusion of physical pathology (especially urinary infection), parental reassurance and the institution of a behavioural programme (star chart and/or bell and pad). Tricyclic antidepressants are effective (mechanism unclear), but relapse is frequent when they are discontinued. Anticholinergic drugs (oxybutinin) and synthetic antidiuretic hormone (desmopressin) are increasingly used. Ninety per cent resolve by adolescence.

Encopresis involves the deposition of a normal or near normal stool in inappropriate places in the presence of normal bowel control. Most children are faecally continent by the age of 4 years. Prevalence is about 2% in boys and 1% in girls at age 8 years. Encopresis may reflect anger (with deposits positioned to cause maximum distress) or regression in children unable to cope with the increasing independence expected of them. Voluntary faecal retention with subsequent overflow is present in some cases. Physical disorder (e.g. Hirschsprung's disease) and other causes for constipation or pain on defecation must be ruled out. Encopresis is associated with emotional disturbance and other psychiatric disorders (although none is characteristic) and intelligence is usually average or below. There may be underlying parental marital conflicts, punitive potty training and/or sexual abuse. Treatment aims both to restore normal bowel habit and to improve parent/child relationships. Parents should be encouraged to ignore the soiling and in particular not to punish the child. More specific treatments include behaviour modification (e.g. star chart) and family therapy. Drug treatments are of very little use, except the use of laxatives if constipation is present. Ninety per cent improve within 1 year and almost all cases resolve by adolescence. Associated conduct disorder may, however, persist.

Hyperkinetic disorders

The core hyperkinetic syndrome (also called attention-deficit hyperactivity disorder [ADHD]) is characterized by an early onset (usually 3–8 years) of short attention span, distractibility, overactivity and impulsivity which lasts longer than 6 months. It is more common in boys (male/female ratio is 3:1), may be 'pervasive' (both at home and school) or 'situational' and is often associated with antisocial behaviour, language delay or clumsiness. It is less commonly recognized in the UK (<1%) than in the USA (7%), although this probably reflects UK usage of a narrower concept of ADHD. ADHD frequently coexists with conduct disorder, anxiety, depression and SRR. Comorbidity predicts a poorer prognosis. Children with comorbid ADHD and conduct disorder are at particular risk of substance disorders in adolescence; severe forms are often associated with low intelligence, particularly in the context of brain damage (cerebral palsy, epilepsy). Other aetiological factors may include genetic loading, social adversity, parental alcohol abuse, dietary constituents (lead, tartrazine) and exposure to tranquillizers. Treatment approaches include behaviour modification, exclusion diets and (paradoxically) stimulants such as methylphenidate (which has recently become available in slow-release form). Tricyclic antidepressants, clonidine, bupropion, antipsychotics and atomoxetine are also sometimes used. Hyperactivity usually lessens by adolescence, although learning difficulties often persist and there is an excess of adult antisocial behaviour. There is increasing recognition that some childhood ADHD may be part of an affective (manic) disorder.

Psychotic disorders

Psychoses of childhood are rare. The most important are the childhood *schizophrenias* which may be acute in onset (carrying a better prognosis) or have a prodrome of apparent developmental delay. As in adolescence and adulthood, there is a genetic predisposition and the presentation is with hallucinations, delusions and thought disorder, but with a greater preponderance of motility disturbance, particularly catatonia. Antipsychotics are the mainstay of treatment. Mania was thought not to occur before adolescence but is now increasingly recognized in the post-pubertal years. The *disintegrative psychoses* of childhood are characterized by normal initial development (to age 4 years) and the subsequent onset of a dementia with social, language and motor regression with prominent stereotypies. The aetiology includes infections (especially subacute sclerosing panencephalitis) and neurometabolic disorders. Prognosis is poor.

23 The psychiatry of adolescence

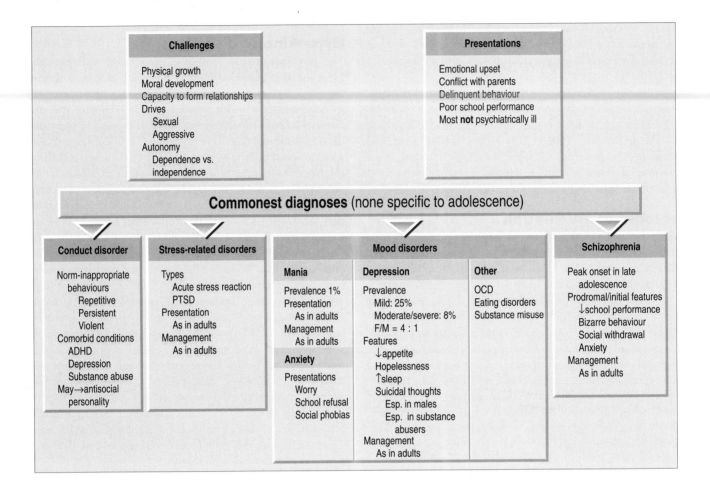

Challenges	Presentations

Physical growth
Moral development
Capacity to form relationships
Drives
  Sexual
  Aggressive
Autonomy
  Dependence vs.
  independence
	Emotional upset
	Conflict with parents
	Delinquent behaviour
	Poor school performance
	Most **not** psychiatrically ill

Commonest diagnoses (none specific to adolescence)

Conduct disorder

Norm-inappropriate
  behaviours
    Repetitive
    Persistent
    Violent
Comorbid conditions
  ADHD
  Depression
  Substance abuse
May→antisocial
  personality

Stress-related disorders

Types
  Acute stress reaction
  PTSD
Presentation
  As in adults
Management
  As in adults

Mood disorders

Mania	Depression	Other

Prevalence 1%
Presentation
  As in adults
Management
  As in adults
 	
Anxiety
 	
Presentations
  Worry
  School refusal
  Social phobias
	Prevalence
	  Mild: 25%
	  Moderate/severe: 8%
	  F/M = 4 : 1
	Features
	  ↓appetite
	  Hopelessness
	  ↑sleep
	  Suicidal thoughts
	    Esp. in males
	    Esp. in substance
	      abusers
	Management
	  As in adults
		OCD
		Eating disorders
		Substance misuse

Schizophrenia

Peak onset in late
  adolescence
Prodromal/initial features
  ↓school performance
  Bizarre behaviour
  Social withdrawal
  Anxiety
Management
  As in adults

Adolescence stretches from the onset of puberty to the attainment of full physical maturity. It encompasses considerable changes, including sudden physical growth, surging sexual and aggressive drives (with associated uncertainties about sexual role, adequacy and identity) and the transition to autonomy and separation from parents (and associated dependence/independence conflict). Moral values may be expected to crystallize and self-esteem to grow. Conflicts between individual development and societal expectations may arise, and peer-group pressures and influences are crucial. Added challenges include career choice and commitment to work. The capacity for lasting relationships develops in adolescence; difficulties in forming relationships may emerge. Although adolescence is often a time of turmoil, true psychiatric disturbance is relatively rare. No psychiatric diagnoses are specific to adolescence; most adult and child psychiatric disorders are seen, often modified by the patient's developmental stage.

Psychiatric assessment in adolescence

Common presentations of psychiatric disorder in adolescence include emotional upset, identity issues, conflict with parents, delinquent behaviour and poor school performance. Psychiatric assessment presents a number of challenges. A developmental perspective is crucial, since both level of functioning and apparent 'disorders' must be set against developmental norms. Patients often do not acknowledge their own problems, and referral by parent or school may itself be a source of conflict and distress. Trust and rapport must be built up slowly in the face of resentment, suspicion and the fear of being thought 'mad'. The patient's right to confidentiality must be respected, particularly in the context of sexual abuse. Involving the family is important not only to provide corroborative evidence (the patient's own account often being inadequate or even falsified), but also to build up a picture of the family dynamics that may be crucial in both aetiology and management. A full account of earlier development is particularly important since many adolescent disorders have clear childhood antecedents. Although a number of structured interview schedules and behaviour ratings are available, the diagnostic process is the same as in adults, with most patients having disorders within the DSM or ICD classifications. Comorbidity is, however, even more common than in adults.

Conduct disorder

Conduct disorder (CD) may emerge in adolescence or, if already established, be exacerbated. The essential feature is of conduct violating age-appropriate societal norms. The behaviours are repetitive, persistent and often violent; bullying, mugging, shoplifting, theft, property damage or even armed robbery are common. CD is associated with low socio-economic class. 'Solitary' and 'group' patterns of CD are described. Substance abuse (see below), attention-deficit hyperactivity disorder (ADHD) and depression (see below) often coexist with CD. Coexistent ADHD worsens the prognosis of CD. About one-third of adolescents with CD develop adult antisocial personality disorder, with continuing violent recidivism. Treatment may involve individual and/or family psychotherapy and appropriate management of comorbid conditions. If problems are severe, medication may be used cautiously. Lithium, haloperidol and carbamazepine may reduce aggressive behaviour. Selective serotonin reuptake inhibitors (SSRIs) may reduce impulsivity, irritability and lability of mood.

Eating disorders

Anorexia nervosa (AN) and bulimia nervosa (BN) are each found in about 1% of adolescents. AN has its peak prevalence in adolescence, and if mild may be difficult to distinguish from age-appropriate preoccupation with dieting. Adolescent-onset BN is increasingly common. Obesity is also common in adolescence (prevalence 20–30%). These conditions are discussed in Chapter 11.

Substance abuse

Experimentation with psychoactive substances (tobacco, alcohol, illegal drugs) is common in adolescence, reflecting both adolescent rebellion and the easy availability of the substances. In most cases, there is no lasting harm. Family and social adversity, vulnerable personality, peer pressure and associated CD or depression can contribute to the aetiology of adolescent substance abuse. The hallmarks of problematic abuse are abrupt deterioration in school performance (truancy, low grades, poor discipline), social difficulties (lawbreaking, fights, apparent personality change), slow movements, lethargy, lack of motivation, slurred speech, drowsiness, lack of concentration, absenteeism from school and an unexplained deterioration in physical health. The patient usually denies any problems, and information from school or friends may be vital. There may be other features of CD, and depression is frequent. The rise in adolescent suicide is largely accounted for by substance abusers, and suicide risk must be assessed.

Mood disorders

Mild episodes of depression (characterized by loneliness and low self-esteem) occur in 25% of adolescents and moderate or severe depression in about 8%. Depression is about four times more common in adolescent girls than in adolescent boys. Clinical features are essentially the same as in adults, but poor appetite, weight loss and feelings of hopelessness may be more prominent than overt sadness; sleep is more often prolonged than disrupted. Suicidal thoughts (and minor acts of deliberate self-harm) are common; risk of actual suicide (particularly in boys and where there is coexistent substance abuse) must be considered. Anxiety, eating disorders, substance abuse and ADHD all frequently coexist with depression in adolescence. Intervention may include family therapy and individual psychotherapy (particularly cognitive–behaviour; see Chapter 32). Antidepressants (see Chapter 33) are particularly indicated where biological features are prominent.

Mania has a prevalence of up to 1% in adolescence; the presentation and management principles are similar to those in adults. Substance abuse and schizophrenia are the main differential diagnoses.

Anxiety, stress-related disorders

Anxiety most frequently presents as overwhelming, non-specific worry and repeated demands for reassurance. School refusal (as opposed to truancy) may arise both from specific school-related phobias and from separation anxiety. Social phobias, characterized by avoiding contact with strangers, are also seen. Milder forms may respond to reassurance and advice (to adolescent, parents and school) on coping strategies; in more serious cases, response to relaxation and desensitization is usually favourable. Anxiety may also arise in response to stress, with both acute stress reaction and post-traumatic stress disorder (PTSD) having similar characteristics to their adult counterparts. Management of stress-related anxiety is on similar principles to those used in adults, but the emphasis is more strongly on a behavioural or psychotherapeutic approach, with tranquillizers being resorted to only rarely. SSRIs may be useful in social phobias.

Obsessive–compulsive disorder (OCD)

Mild obsessionality is common in adolescence; true OCD may show prominent obsessional slowness and behaviour sufficiently bizarre to resemble schizophrenia. Resistance to the thoughts and behaviours may be absent. Tourette's syndrome may coexist. Treatment usually involves both behavioural treatments, for example modelling and response prevention, and serotonin-reuptake blocking antidepressants (clomipramine, SSRIs). OCD usually continues into adult life.

Schizophrenia

The peak age of onset of schizophrenia is in late adolescence. Presentation is usually with deteriorating school performance; clinical features are otherwise as in adult life. In younger adolescents, initial presentation is often with bizarre behaviour, social withdrawal and anxiety, with only fleeting first-rank symptoms. The differential diagnosis includes organic states, affective psychosis, drug-induced psychosis, adolescent crises and schizoid personality. Antipsychotics (despite frequent sensitivity to sedative and extrapyramidal side-effects) and rehabilitation are the mainstays of management.

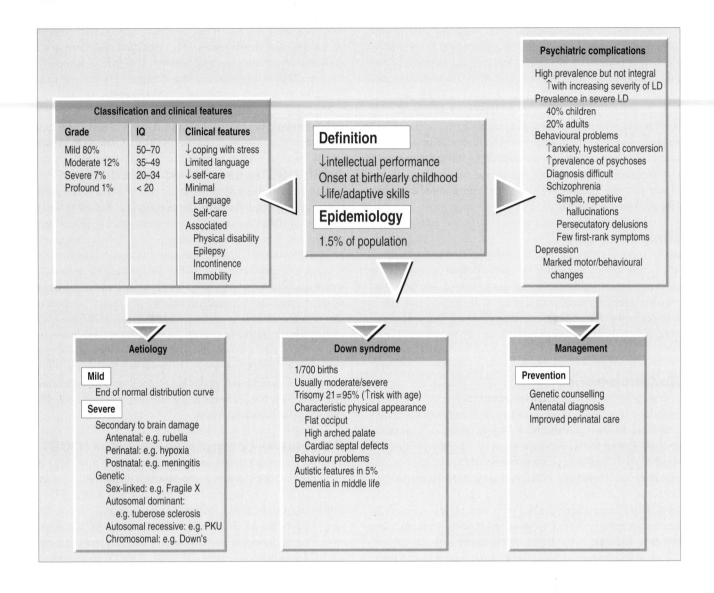

Classification and clinical features

Grade	IQ	Clinical features
Mild 80%	50–70	↓coping with stress
Moderate 12%	35–49	Limited language
Severe 7%	20–34	↓self-care
Profound 1%	< 20	Minimal
		Language
		Self-care
		Associated
		Physical disability
		Epilepsy
		Incontinence
		Immobility

Definition

↓intellectual performance
Onset at birth/early childhood
↓life/adaptive skills

Epidemiology

1.5% of population

Psychiatric complications

High prevalence but not integral
↑with increasing severity of LD
Prevalence in severe LD
40% children
20% adults
Behavioural problems
↑anxiety, hysterical conversion
↑prevalence of psychoses
Diagnosis difficult
Schizophrenia
Simple, repetitive
hallucinations
Persecutatory delusions
Few first-rank symptoms
Depression
Marked motor/behavioural
changes

Aetiology

Mild
End of normal distribution curve

Severe
Secondary to brain damage
Antenatal: e.g. rubella
Perinatal: e.g. hypoxia
Postnatal: e.g. meningitis
Genetic
Sex-linked: e.g. Fragile X
Autosomal dominant:
e.g. tuberose sclerosis
Autosomal recessive: e.g. PKU
Chromosomal: e.g. Down's

Down syndrome

1/700 births
Usually moderate/severe
Trisomy 21 = 95% (↑risk with age)
Characteristic physical appearance
Flat occiput
High arched palate
Cardiac septal defects
Behaviour problems
Autistic features in 5%
Dementia in middle life

Management

Prevention
Genetic counselling
Antenatal diagnosis
Improved perinatal care

Definition

Learning disability (LD; referred to as mental retardation in current classificatory systems) has three main components: low intellectual performance; onset at birth or in early childhood; reduced life/adaptive skills.

Classification and clinical features

LD can be conceptualized in terms of the primary impairment that causes it, the consequent disability and any resultant social handicap (including family difficulties). Intellectual impairment is classified as mild (IQ 50–70); moderate (35–49); severe (20–34) and profound (<20). Mild LD is not usually associated with abnormalities in appearance or behaviour; language, sensory and motor abnormalities are slight or absent. The problem is usually not apparent until school age. Adults with mild LD may have difficulty in coping with stress and often need support with more complex areas of social functioning, such as parenting and handling finance. The

majority are, however, able to live independently in the community and sustain some employment. People with moderate LD usually have limited but useful language. Severe and profound LD is associated with very limited verbal and self-care skills; associated physical disabilities/problems (epilepsy in 33%, incontinence in about 10%, inability to walk in about 15%) are very common. Communication may be facilitated by non-verbal techniques such as pointing, tagging or signing. LD is present in about 1.5% of the population. Eighty per cent of cases have mild LD, about 12% moderate and 7% are severely affected. Only 1% is profoundly affected. The prevalence of LD has not fallen despite recent reductions in the incidence of severe LD. This reflects concurrent improvements in prevention (see below) and survival.

Psychiatric disorder (including behavioural disturbance) has a high prevalence in people with LD but is not integral to it. Behavioural disturbance is commoner with increasing severity of LD, occurring in up to 40% of children and 20% of adults with severe

LD. This may include purposeless or self-injurious behaviour, aggression, or inappropriate sexual behaviour such as masturbation in public.

Mild LD is not usually associated with specific causes and represents the bottom end of a normal distribution curve for IQ; there is a considerable genetic contribution reflecting the high heritability of IQ in general. The close correlation between low parental and low child IQ is, however, due in part to (potentially reversible) social and educational deprivation. More severe LD is usually related to specific brain damage. Causes may be antenatal (genetic, infective, hypoxic, toxic or related to maternal disease such as toxaemia of pregnancy), perinatal (prematurity, birth hypoxia, intracerebral bleed) or postnatal (infection, injury [particularly non-accidental], malnutrition, hormonal, metabolic, toxic, epileptic). Genetic causes may be chromosomal, e.g. Down, Klinefelter and Turner's syndromes, X-linked (Fragile X, Lesch–Nyhan), autosomal dominant (tuberose sclerosis, neurofibromatosis) and autosomal recessive, the latter usually associated with specific metabolic disorders such as phenylketonuria (PKU).

Fragile X is the second commonest cause of LD, accounting for 8% of males with LD. Physical signs include large head and ears, connective tissue disorders and mitral valve prolapse. Psychiatric features include abnormal speech, impulsivity and hyperactivity. Four per cent have autistic features. The most important antenatal infective agents are toxoplasma, rubella and cytomegalovirus. Perinatal injury frequently causes cerebral palsy (which may be associated with normal intelligence) as well as LD. Autism (see Chapter 22) is usually, although not invariably, associated with LD.

Down syndrome (DS)

DS is the commonest specific cause of LD, affecting about 1/700 births. The LD is usually moderate or severe, although only mild LD is present in 15%. Individuals with DS may be stubborn, oppositional and impulsive. Autistic features are present in 5%. In 95% of cases there is trisomy of chromosome 21, risk of which increases with increasing maternal age (1/50 births with maternal age >45 years). In the remainder, DS is the result of translocation of chromosome 21 material; parents and siblings may be carriers. DS is associated with several physical abnormalities including flat occiput, oblique palpebral fissures, small mouth with high arched palate and broad hands with a single transverse palmar crease. Cardiac septal defects are common and used to result in high early mortality; they are now often corrected. Hypothyroidism is common. Post-mortem studies of people with DS indicate that those surviving beyond the age of 50 years invariably develop neuropathological changes akin to Alzheimer's disease (see Chapter 18); clinical dementia is, however, not always apparent in life but develops in at least 50% of cases

Psychiatric illness (dual diagnosis)

Challenging behaviours are common in both children and adults with LD and are often related to psychiatric disorder. Making specific psychiatric diagnoses is, however, difficult (particularly in people with moderate or severe LD) because of coexisting language deficits. Studies using appropriately structured interviews, detailed behavioural observation and carer data reveal that the prevalence of several psychiatric disorders is increased. Rates are higher in institutional than in community populations. Schizophrenia has a prevalence of 3% and usually presents with simple and repetitive hallucinations and unelaborated, usually persecutory, delusions; these usually lack the complexity of first-rank symptoms (see Chapter 3). The diagnosis of depression rests more on motor and behavioural changes (reduced sleep, retardation, tearfulness, etc.) than verbal expressions of depressed mood; similarly, mania usually presents as overactive and/or irritable behaviour. Phobic anxiety and hysterical conversion symptoms are both common as are psychological reactions to adverse life events. These are, however, often not recognized as such by carers. Genetic, organic (particularly epilepsy), psychological (frustration) and social factors such as family tension, may all contribute to the excess of psychiatric problems associated with LD.

Prevention

Prevention of LD may be attempted before birth through genetic counselling and antenatal diagnosis; in particular, DS may be detected by amniocentesis or chorionic villus sampling, with the option of termination of pregnancy. Improved perinatal care reduces the risk of brain injury, and early detection of hormonal or metabolic problems (myxoedema, phenylketonuria) may allow treatment before LD sets in. There is some evidence that educational intervention in children of mothers with mild LD may enhance their educational performance (although not necessarily their IQ) and reduce the risk of conduct disorder.

Management

The movement towards community care has enabled the great majority of people with LD to live in a domestic rather than an institutional setting, usually with their families. Support is provided by the general practitioner (GP) and through educational and social services. Educational support for children with mild LD is usually within mainstream schools; in adult life they may need continuing support to hold down open-market jobs. Further training may enable adults with moderate LD to work in appropriate sheltered settings; a small minority (with severe or profound LD and, usually, associated behavioural problems) nonetheless need residential care. Specialist support provided by multidisiplinary community teams involves coordination of local services, assessment of individuals and management of any concurrent mental illness identified, as well as social skills and problem training, and support with finances and accommodation. The former requires a high index of suspicion and similar treatment principles to those in patients of normal intelligence, including appropriate use of psychotropic medication and a multidisciplinary approach to treatment including accessible information and communication techniques, rehabilitation and work with families or paid carers. Challenging behaviour is usually dealt with by psychological means with a greater emphasis on behavioural techniques and on enriching the individual's milieu.

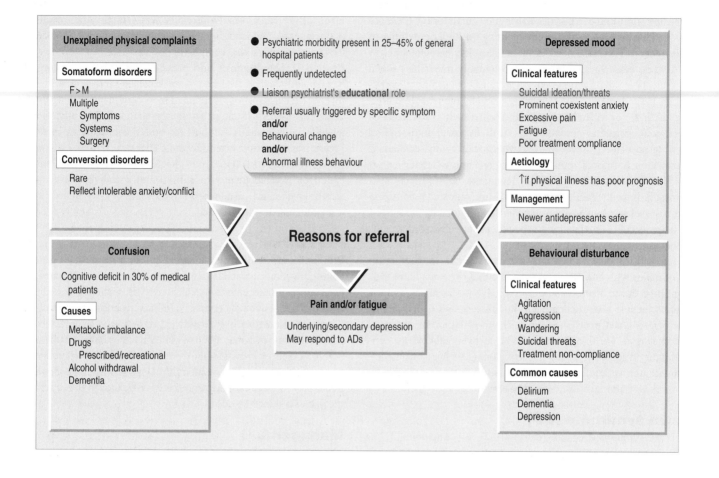

Reasons for referral

- Psychiatric morbidity present in 25–45% of general hospital patients
- Frequently undetected
- Liaison psychiatrist's **educational** role
- Referral usually triggered by specific symptom **and/or** Behavioural change **and/or** Abnormal illness behaviour

Unexplained physical complaints

Somatoform disorders

F > M
Multiple
  Symptoms
  Systems
  Surgery

Conversion disorders

Rare
Reflect intolerable anxiety/conflict

Confusion

Cognitive deficit in 30% of medical patients

Causes

Metabolic imbalance
Drugs
  Prescribed/recreational
Alcohol withdrawal
Dementia

Pain and/or fatigue

Underlying/secondary depression
May respond to ADs

Depressed mood

Clinical features

Suicidal ideation/threats
Prominent coexistent anxiety
Excessive pain
Fatigue
Poor treatment compliance

Aetiology

↑if physical illness has poor prognosis

Management

Newer antidepressants safer

Behavioural disturbance

Clinical features

Agitation
Aggression
Wandering
Suicidal threats
Treatment non-compliance

Common causes

Delirium
Dementia
Depression

Consultation–liaison psychiatry refers to the practice of psychiatry on general hospital wards or by the joint care and management of people with both medical and psychological difficulties by physicians and psychiatrists. The narrower concept of 'psychosomatic disorders' originally referred to somatic conditions in which there was a structural change or lesion in a target end organ: the aetiology was primarily psychological, such as chronic stress, and the effects were mediated via the hypothalamic/pituitary axis. Such conditions would include peptic ulceration, asthma, hypertension and certain types of dermatitis. It is now recognized that psychiatric morbidity (consisting mainly of organic disorders, depression and anxiety) is present in a high (25–45%) proportion of medical and surgical patients, largely irrespective of their primary diagnosis. This reflects both the psychiatric disturbances secondary to physical illness and the increased physical vulnerability that psychiatric difficulties impart. Psychiatric disorder may be important in mediating the established link between adverse life events and physical illness. In addition, abnormalities of personality may predispose to specific physical illness. Aggressiveness, hostility driving and competitive striving ('type A behaviours') may, for example, predispose to myocardial infarction, and emotional suppression, unassertiveness and overcompliance to cancer.

Rates of referral by physicians and surgeons to the liaison psychiatrist are generally low. Referrals are not always for a specific suspected psychiatric illness. They may be triggered by behavioural disturbance, where real physical symptoms are exaggerated or denied (abnormal illness behaviour), or by failure to find a clear cause for persistent physical symptoms. Underreferral may reflect not only underdetection but physicians' belief that emotional disorders are simply an understandable response to physical illness, and fear that psychiatric referral will itself generate anxiety or resentment.

The review below will concentrate on principles of managing problems arising in individual medical or surgical patients for whom the liaison psychiatrist may need to provide follow-up as well as acute assessment. The wider brief of liaison psychiatry is educational, in encouraging awareness of psychological aspects of medical illness and thereby enabling earlier detection of individual problems.

Coexistent psychiatric disorders in medical or surgical patients

Organic mental disorder must always be considered in any hospital patient presenting with alteration of behaviour or mood, particularly where there is evidence of cognitive impairment. As many as 30% of acute medical patients have some cognitive deficit, reflecting in part the vulnerability of the aged both to cognitive and physical disorders. Delirium (see Chapter 17) is characterized by impaired attention, clouding of conciousness, fluctuating conciousness, labile affect, disorientation and perceptual disturbance. Common underlying causes in medical patients (usually reversible if identified in time) include metabolic imbalance (reflecting major body system failure), stroke, drugs (both prescribed and recreational) and alcohol withdrawal. Dementia (see Chapter 18) may first become apparent in the setting of acute physical illness, as patients reveal their inability to learn to cope in a novel environment and without family support. Dementia is associated with increased length of hospital stay and its early detection may facilitate appropriate discharge planning.

Depressed mood may trigger psychiatric referral of a medical patient. Such depression often has associated *anxiety symptoms* and may represent an adjustment disorder (see Chapter 8), particularly where the concurrent physical illness has a poor prognosis in terms of chronicity (e.g. diabetes), level of incapacitation or life expectancy. Supportive psychotherapy may be helpful in coming to terms with the consequences of illness. Depressive symptoms may become severe and render patients suicidal or non-compliant with treatment. Antidepressants may be beneficial, but the potential cardiotoxicity of tricyclics (as well as the risk of anticholinergic confusion) is particularly important in this vulnerable group, and newer antidepressants (e.g. selective serotonin reuptake inhibitors [SSRIs]) may be preferred. Structural brain disease or injury can also cause organic mood disorders, the best known example being the link between stroke (particularly following left anterior infarcts) and depression.

Patients with *pre-existing psychiatric illness* may require urgent medical or surgical management. This is particularly likely in the context of alcohol or substance abuse, with their well-established medical complications, and in patients with established depression or schizophrenia who attempt suicide which may lead to multiple injuries. Such patients will need continued psychiatric management with careful monitoring of their mental state under stressful circumstances. This should also include support and reassurance to medical staff. Particular attention should be paid to possible interactions between psychotropic drugs and any new medical condition or treatment.

Other reasons for psychiatric referral

Psychiatric referral is often triggered by chronic physical complaints for which no organic cause can be found. Rarely, this reflects a *conversion disorder* in which intolerable psychic anxiety or stress is 'converted' into more acceptable and bearable physical symptoms about which the patient seems relatively unconcerned ('*la belle*

indifference'). The key to management is detection of the underlying conflict and reconnecting the patient to feelings associated with it. This may require specialized techniques such as hypnosis or abreaction.

More common are the group of *somatoform disorders*. Somatization disorder (sometimes known as Briquet's syndrome) is much commoner in women than in men, and is characterized by complaints involving multiple body systems, starting before the age of 30 years, and often resulting in multiple operations despite the absence of organic disorder. Related conditions include *hypochondriacal disorder* (non-delusional preoccupation with the possibility of serious illness such as cancer, heart disease or acquired immunodeficiency syndrome [AIDS]), *somatoform autonomic disorder* (with predominant autonomic dysfunction such as sweating, palpitations or hyperventilation) and persistent somatoform pain disorder (chronic pain without organic basis).

Management of these conditions involves ensuring that there really is no organic basis, and exploring with the patient (and the family) any 'secondary gain' (such as sympathy or avoidance of family conflict) that might be encouraging symptom maintenance or the 'sick role'.

Pain may trigger psychiatric referral even without clear evidence of somatoform disorder. Depression may underlie such pain or result from it, particularly if organically caused pain is inadequately treated for fear of causing opiate dependence. Chronic pain may respond to antidepressants (especially SSRIs) even in the absence of clear-cut depression, and often at doses too low to be antidepressant. Similar considerations apply to *fatigue*, a feature common to many physical and psychiatric illnesses. In particular, the combination of exhaustion after minimal physical activity, poor concentration and muscle tenderness which constitutes myalgic encephalomyelitis shares many features with depression and may respond to antidepressants.

Psychiatric advice may be requested to deal with *behavioural problems* such as agitation, aggressivity, wandering, deliberate self-harm (especially in the Accident and Emergency department) and non-compliance with treatment. Patients presenting with such behavioural disturbance frequently have delirium (which must be excluded or its underlying cause identified and treated as a matter of urgency) or dementia. Suicidal threats or gestures may also cause considerable anxiety in ward nursing staff, who may need advice in both assessment and management of suicide risk (see Chapter 7). Multidisciplinary discussion of behavioural problems can often identify triggers to undesirable behaviour and help ward staff find ways of defusing provocative situations. Appropriate advice may also be needed on the use of tranquillizing drugs and on the legal implications of ignoring (or respecting) patients' refusal of treatment or desire to leave hospital against medical advice.

Psychiatry in the community

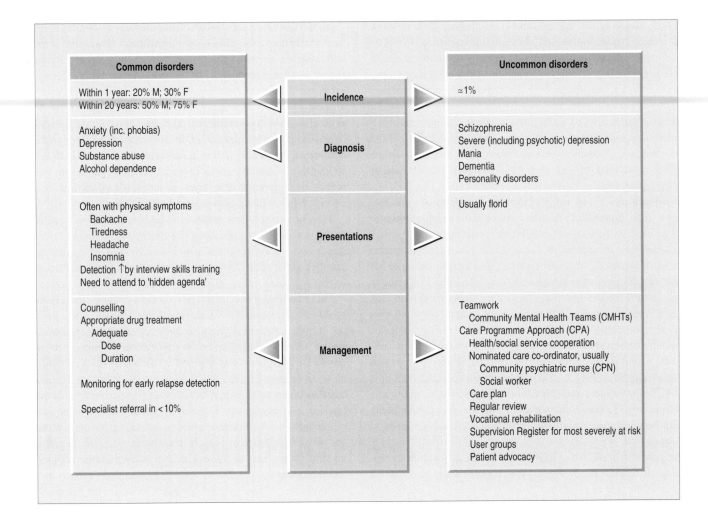

Common disorders		Uncommon disorders

Common disorders		Uncommon disorders
Within 1 year: 20% M; 30% F Within 20 years: 50% M; 75% F	**Incidence**	≈1%
Anxiety (inc. phobias) Depression Substance abuse Alcohol dependence	**Diagnosis**	Schizophrenia Severe (including psychotic) depression Mania Dementia Personality disorders

Often with physical symptoms
   Backache
   Tiredness
   Headache
   Insomnia
Detection ↑by interview skills training
Need to attend to 'hidden agenda'
	Presentations	Usually florid

Counselling
Appropriate drug treatment
   Adequate
      Dose
      Duration
 	
Monitoring for early relapse detection
 	
Specialist referral in <10%
	Management	Teamwork
		   Community Mental Health Teams (CMHTs)
		Care Programme Approach (CPA)
		   Health/social service cooperation
		   Nominated care co-ordinator, usually
		      Community psychiatric nurse (CPN)
		      Social worker
		   Care plan
		   Regular review
		   Vocational rehabilitation
		   Supervision Register for most severely at risk
		   User groups
		   Patient advocacy

The traditional model of caring for patients in the hospital or in out-patient clinics is only one part of a comprehensive mental health care system. Most patients with disabling psychological illness, particularly where this is relatively mild, are dealt with in a primary care setting (if their illness is detected at all). At the other extreme, there has been a considerable shift in locus of care for people with severe and chronic psychiatric illness from the psychiatric hospital into the community. This chapter reviews the delivery of community psychiatric care.

Psychiatry in primary care

Community surveys in the UK and USA suggest that about 25% of the population aged between 18 and 65 years will experience significant psychiatric morbidity within a 1-year period, women outnumbering men by a factor of about 1.5. Over 20 years, the proportion rises to 75% of women and 50% of men. The majority of such illnesses consist of anxiety disorders (including phobias and adjustment reactions) and depression (many patients having features of both). A further important group will have substance abuse (including alcohol) problems. A few will have chronic psychotic or personality problems; new psychoses (schizophrenic or affective)

are relatively rare. In the elderly, the total prevalence of psychiatric illness is particularly high because of the age-associated rise in prevalence of dementia.

In the UK, virtually the whole population is registered with a general practitioner (GP), and psychiatric morbidity doubles the likelihood of GP consultation. About one-third of patients with significant psychiatric illness will, however, not be recognized by the GP as psychiatrically ill. Patient factors influencing non-detection (which is associated with poor prognosis) include attitude to illness (e.g. not accepting it as psychiatric or as treatable) and to the GP (perceived as not sympathetic or understanding). GP training, attitudes and time available for consultation may also contribute. Detection rates may be increased by interview-skills training, encouraging such factors as eye contact, sensitivity to non-verbal cues and avoidance of exclusive concentration on the presenting complaint at the expense of any 'hidden agenda', of past or chronic problems and of the social and family background. Detection of depression may further be increased by awareness of its frequently somatic presentation (e.g. tiredness, headache, backache, insomnia).

Only about one-eighth of cases detected will be referred to

psychiatrists. The decision to refer may reflect the GP's confidence in managing psychiatric illness, the patient's wishes and the accessibility of the psychiatric service, as well as the severity and duration of the patient's illness.

The challenge of primary care psychiatry is to ensure recognition and optimal care for the submerged iceberg of psychiatric morbidity. Minor anxiety disorders respond to counselling (from practice-based counsellors or psychologists) and depressions to antidepressants or, where available, brief cognitive or problem-solving psychotherapy.

Psychiatrists are increasingly involved in GP surgeries, seeing individual patients, giving management advice and teaching GPs and practice staff (particularly practice nurses) about detection and management of common psychiatric conditions. This might, for example, involve advice on psychological management and on when to refer, as well as encouragement to use drug treatments appropriately. In particular, GPs frequently administer antidepressants at suboptimal doses and for too short a time for acute response to occur or (if patients do recover) to minimize risk of relapse.

Community care of severe psychiatric illness

In the past 40 years, there has been a substantial move away from the hospital as the focus of treatment for severe psychiatric illness. Acute admissions have become fewer and briefer, and continuing care beds have dwindled by more than 50%. Factors involved include the effectiveness of psychotropic drugs, an ideological commitment to the closure of asylum-type psychiatric hospitals and reductions in bed numbers as a cost-cutting exercise.

Closing psychiatric beds is no guarantee of adequate community care. Good community care is usually just as expensive as institutional care, but if adequately resourced can avoid institutionalization and has been shown to achieve high standards both in symptom control and in patient and family satisfaction. In contrast, poor quality 'cheap' community care can result in gross failure, with increasing numbers of homeless people suffering from severe, untreated and unmonitored mental illness. Good community care should be locally accessible. Psychiatrists and community nurses may work from GP surgeries (see above) or in community mental health centres. Patients unable to live independently may be cared for by family or friends (who may themselves need support from services if they are to provide this care). This may not be appropriate since close family contact where there is a lot of 'friction' (high expressed emotion) may increase the risk of schizophrenic relapse. Professional support may be provided in supported accommodation projects such as group homes or hostels. These are usually run by social service or voluntary organizations; the amount of professional support can vary from 24-h nursing staff to peripatetic mental health workers visiting two or three times per week. The assessment of an individual's level of function in terms of activities of daily living (such as personal hygiene, shopping, budgeting, cooking and cleaning) as well as their attitude towards and compliance with medication is therefore very important in deciding what level of support they will need to live successfully in the community and for them to avoid relapse and return to hospital. Due to the complex nature of the social security benefit system, rehabilitating people back to work can be problematic. However, finding appropriate employment is a goal of many community services for people with severe mental health problems. Meaningful occupation such as 'sheltered work' and day care at day centres can be important for those whose disabilities prevent them from achieving mainstream employment. Giving structure to people's lives and increasing their social support networks are very important in the maintenance of successful community rehabilitation, and vocational rehabilitation aims to achieve this. Increasingly, occupational therapy focuses on linking people with mainstream vocational services such as college courses and training in various skills in preparation for open employment. Vocational rehabilitation has been identified as a crucial factor in enabling patients to lead fulfilling lives and is highly associated with patient satisfaction.

Risk of relapse in the community must always be considered, with careful monitoring and continued medication where appropriate. The community care coordinator has an important role in monitoring patients' clinical state and providing practical support as well as monitoring medication compliance and, where appropriate community mental health nurses will administer depot injections. Other factors in relapse prevention include avoidance of stress and excessive alcohol or illicit drug use.

Detailed care plans for individual patients are developed and reviewed on a regular basis through the Care Programme Approach (CPA). These are a statutory requirement for all patients under the care of Community Mental Health Teams and often involve cooperation between several services (primarily the health and social services but also housing, GP, family, etc.). This implies considerable negotiation and coordination, with full case-note documentation of agreed care plans. The nomination of a 'care coordinator' (who may be a social worker, nurse, occupational therapist or psychologist) is crucial to the delivery of the care package. In the UK this approach was formalized within the 1991 Community Care Act, which stipulates that health and social services in particular should agree and monitor care plans for the more severely ill patients. A further important element is involvement of the family and of the patient in the development of the care plan. The growth of 'user groups' and of the 'patient advocacy' movement has helped encourage this.

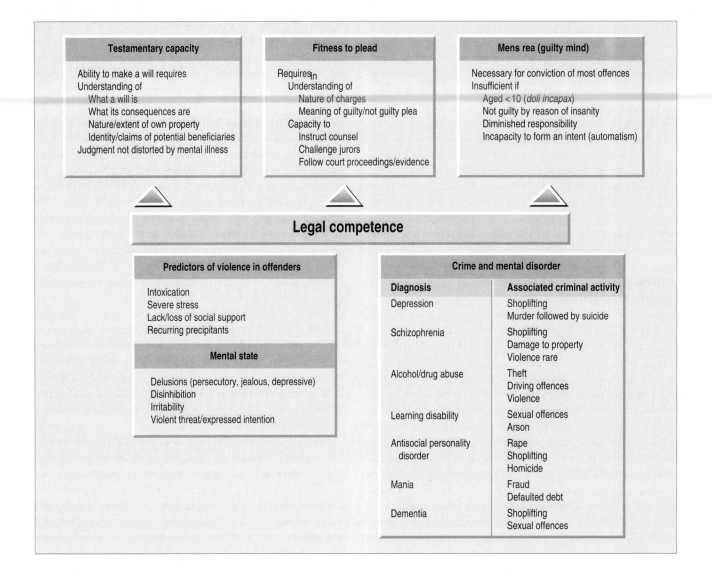

Testamentary capacity

Ability to make a will requires
Understanding of
  What a will is
  What its consequences are
  Nature/extent of own property
  Identity/claims of potential beneficiaries
Judgment not distorted by mental illness

Fitness to plead

Requires
Understanding of
  Nature of charges
  Meaning of guilty/not guilty plea
Capacity to
  Instruct counsel
  Challenge jurors
  Follow court proceedings/evidence

Mens rea (guilty mind)

Necessary for conviction of most offences
Insufficient if
  Aged < 10 (*doli incapax*)
  Not guilty by reason of insanity
  Diminished responsibility
  Incapacity to form an intent (automatism)

Legal competence

Predictors of violence in offenders

Intoxication
Severe stress
Lack/loss of social support
Recurring precipitants

Mental state

Delusions (persecutory, jealous, depressive)
Disinhibition
Irritability
Violent threat/expressed intention

Crime and mental disorder

Diagnosis	Associated criminal activity
Depression	Shoplifting
	Murder followed by suicide
Schizophrenia	Shoplifting
	Damage to property
	Violence rare
Alcohol/drug abuse	Theft
	Driving offences
	Violence
Learning disability	Sexual offences
	Arson
Antisocial personality disorder	Rape
	Shoplifting
	Homicide
Mania	Fraud
	Defaulted debt
Dementia	Shoplifting
	Sexual offences

Forensic psychiatry concerns the assessment, treatment and rehabilitation of mentally disordered offenders. The main areas covered are links between *crime and mental disorder*; the assessment of *legal competence* (to form an intent, to plead, to manage financial affairs or to make a will) and of *dangerousness*, and mental health legislation (see Chapter 28), including the disposal and treatment of mentally disordered people.

Crime and mental disorder

Psychiatric illnesses, particularly psychoses and drug- or alcohol-related disorders, are overrepresented in prisoners. This partly reflects a group of urban, homeless, psychiatrically ill, multiple reoffenders; the overall rate of offending by people with a mental illness appears similar to that in the general population. Specific associations have, however, been demonstrated between offences and psychiatric diagnoses.

Patients with *schizophrenia* often commit minor offences such as shoplifting or damage to property. Violence is rare and usually domestic, in response to poor tolerance of family stress. The specific and much publicized link with homicide is usually in the context of florid psychosis secondary to poor treatment compliance.

Depression may be heralded by a minor 'out-of-character' offence (e.g. shoplifting). Depression-related homicide is rare, usually domestic (typically infanticide), often in response to delusions (e.g. believing that the victim is fatally ill and suffering) and frequently followed by suicide. Offences linked to *mania* (fraud, defaulted debt) usually reflect financial irresponsibility.

Alcohol and substance misuse are associated with theft, robbery, assault and homicide. Acute alcohol intoxication weakens inhibitions against offending ('Dutch courage') and is strongly linked with driving offences. Alcohol is often implicated in **morbid or pathological jealousy** (see Chapter 36) which may culminate in spousal homicide.

Dementia is associated with shoplifting (forgetting to pay) and sexual offences (usually reflecting frontal disinhibition). Similarly, subjects with **learning disability** (see Chapter 24) may commit rape or arson. Violent acts may be committed by younger brain-damaged subjects unable to handle stress or frustration.

The link between crime and personality disorder is complex: the link between crime and **antisocial personality disorder** is somewhat circular, since offending may be integral to the diagnosis. Individuals with long-standing paranoid characteristics, people who cannot control their anger and those with severe impulsive and histrionic traits are all more likely than others to offend.

Legal competence

Most mentally ill people retain responsibility for their actions and the capacity to manage their affairs. There are, however, circumstances where the determination of competence is crucial.

Fitness to plead is for a jury to decide and refers to a defendant's competence to mount a defence against charges and consists of the mental capacity to understand the charge, distinguish between guilty and not guilty pleas, instruct lawyers, follow court evidence and challenge jurors. A trial of the facts may nonetheless take place, with acquittal if the facts are not established and flexibility of sentence if proven.

For guilt (of most crimes) to be established, it is necessary to demonstrate that the defendant was 'criminally responsible', possessing the **mens rea** (MR) to commit the offence. MR may be absent by virtue of age, psychiatric illness or automatism and lack of criminal intent (e.g. accidents). Children under 10 years of age cannot be criminally responsible, and for those aged 10–14 years the prosecution must prove MR. Mental disorder is rarely invoked to deny MR; it must be established that the defendant was mentally ill at the time of the offence, resulting in a 'defect of reason', and that consequently he/she could not tell what he/she was doing or know that it was wrong. If successful, the verdict is 'not guilty by reason of insanity'. This theoretically allows some flexibility of sentence, although it usually results in hospital detention. 'Automatism' refers to dissociation between mind and action (e.g. epilepsy, sleepwalking, concussion).

In murder, conviction may be modified to manslaughter on grounds of **diminished responsibility** on the basis of specific 'abnormality of mind' substantially impairing mental responsibility.

Mental disorder (particularly dementia) may impair a person's competence to manage his/her (financial) affairs. Such competence involves understanding of one's property and assets, and any obligations thus incurred. A person may (only while still competent) grant to another a 'Power of Attorney' to manage his/her affairs; this automatically becomes invalid if he/she loses the competence. An 'Enduring Power of Attorney', however, remains valid. The Court of Protection (part of the Supreme Court) can appoint a 'receiver' to manage the affairs of someone who has become incompetent to do so.

Testamentary capacity (competence to make a will; TC) must be present for a will to be valid. It requires a person to understand the act of making a will; to appreciate the extent of his/her property and assets; and to be aware of who might have a reasonable claim on their estate. If the person is mentally ill, TC implies that his/her judgment should not be clouded regarding the will itself. Delusions or hallucinations only impair TC where they are directly relevant to the will (e.g. delusions of poverty).

Predictors of violence in offenders

'Dangerousness' is a judgment based both on the probability of an undesirable act occurring and the potential gravity of that act. Although most psychiatrically disordered people are never dangerous, and most criminally dangerous acts do not take place in the context of mental illness, the assessment of dangerousness is important when planning aftercare. It is important to distinguish between crimes against property and violence against the person. An assessment of dangerousness is not complete unless all relevant past psychiatric and criminal records have been seen. Violent incidents should be accurately documented and not omitted from documentation. The time and date of an incident, the factors preceding it, details of the act itself and the immediate consequences should be accurately recorded at the time. Whilst it is statistically true that the more often an individual has been violent in the past, the more likely a further episode becomes, it is important to be aware that individual factors are the most powerful determinants of behaviour. A first episode of violence can occur in the context of severe stress or a psychotic disorder. Pointers in the mental state examination include expressed violent intentions or threats, irritability, disinhibition, delusions (usually persecutory, jealous or depressive) with potentially dangerous consequences and reluctance to accept treatment An offender who has a past history of violence must be carefully monitored with special reference to recurrence of previous precursors. Other negative factors within current circumstances include intoxication, lack of social support and loss of support. Potential dangerousness may have to be managed by compulsory detention, sometimes long-term. Resource issues should not be allowed to cloud judgments about the management of violence. More general issues of risk assessment and management are discussed in Chapter 29.

Requirements for compulsory detention	⟶	**Mental disorder** **Admission/treatment refused** **Admission necessary for** Patient's health or safety **and/or** Protection of others

Compulsory admission procedures				
MHA Section	**Purpose**	**Recommendation(s)**	**Applicant**	**Duration**
2	Assessment	2 doctors	ASW or NR	28 days
3	Treatment	2 doctors	ASW or NR	6 months
4	Urgent assessment from community	1 doctor	ASW or NR	72 hours
5(2)	Urgent detention of in-patient	1 doctor		72 hours
5(4)	Urgent detention of psychiatric in-patient in absence of doctor	Registered mental nurse		6 hours
136	Removal to place of safety	Police officer		72 hours

Introduction

The MHA, implemented in England and Wales in 1983, is primarily concerned with the care and treatment of mentally disordered patients. The most important sections address compulsory detention by medical recommendation or court order. The MHA is supervised by the Mental Health Act Commission (MHAC) which has also produced a Code of MHA Practice. It should be noted that major changes are envisaged as new Mental Health and Capacity Acts are being fiercely debated (both publicly and within Parliament) at the time of writing.

Definitions

The MHA has four categories of mental disorder (MD): mental illness; mental impairment; severe mental impairment (mental retardation); and psychopathic disorder. The MHA does not, however, provide a definition for mental illness. The MHA does not regard promiscuity, immoral conduct, sexual deviancy or dependence on alcohol or drugs as evidence of MD.

General or non-penal compulsory admission procedures

Compulsory admission procedures ('sectioning') may be implemented only if a patient has MD of sufficient severity to warrant detention in hospital in the interests of his/her own health/safety and/or for the protection/safety of others.

Section 2, admission for assessment (which can include *urgent* treatment) lasts for a maximum of 28 days. Application is made by a social worker 'approved' under the MHA (ASW) or by the nearest relative (NR) on the basis of recommendations by two medical practitioners, one a specialist 'approved' under the MHA Section 12 and the other preferably with 'previous knowledge' of the patient (usually the general practitioner [GP]). Patients may appeal to a Mental Health Review Tribunal (MHRT) within 14 days. MHRTs consist of a lawyer (president), psychiatrist and a lay member (for restricted patients the president is a judge or QC). Patients may be granted legal aid and are able to obtain an independent medical opinion. Near the end of a Section 2 a patient is reassessed with a view to either discharge or detention under Section 3.

Patients may be discharged before the section expires at the discretion of the Responsible Medical Officer (RMO). The MHRT, hospital managers or NR can also implement discharge, although the latter may be barred by the RMO.

Section 3, admission for treatment, lasts 6 months (renewable). The application is by the ASW (after consultation with the NR if possible) or NR. The doctors' recommendation must indicate the nature of the MD and justify three requirements: (i) the patient suffers from MD warranting treatment in hospital; (ii) for mental impairment or psychopathic disorder that such treatment is likely to alleviate or prevent deterioration; and (iii) that such treatment cannot be provided without detention. The patient or NR may apply to the hospital managers or to a MHRT at any time within the first 6 months and once during each subsequent period of renewal. For treatment to continue beyond the first 3 months the patient must either consent (and be attested competent to do so by the RMO) or the treatment plan must be agreed necessary by an independent 'second opinion' psychiatrist nominated by the MHAC. Discharge procedures are as for Section 2. *Section 117* requires that a multi-disciplinary meeting be convened to ensure adequate aftercare for any patient discharged from Section 3. *Section 17* requires that patients on Section 2 and 3 can only be placed on leave subject to the RMO's specific instructions.

Section 4, emergency assessment, lasts 72 hours and is applied for by the ASW or NR. One doctor (preferably with previous knowledge of the patient) makes the recommendation on the grounds that admission (otherwise fulfilling Section 2 requirements) is more urgent than Section 2 procedures would allow.

Section 136 empowers a police constable who finds a person in a public place appearing to suffer from an MD to remove him/her to a 'place of safety' for assessment. It is valid for 72 hours.

Section 135, which lasts 72 hours, empowers a police officer or other authorized person acting on a magistrate's warrant to enter premises in order to remove to a place of safety a person who is suffering from an MD, being ill-treated, neglected, not under proper control or is unable to care for themselves (if living alone).

Section 5(2), for patients already in hospital (receiving any form of treatment), is valid for 72 hours, and is on the recommendation of the doctor in charge of the case or his/her nominated deputy. Patients placed on Section 5(2) must subsequently be assessed for Section 2 or 3.

Section 5(4), a nurse's holding power valid for 6 hours, allows urgent detention of a patient already receiving treatment for MD in hospital when a doctor is not able to attend immediately. Only registered mental nurses (RMNs) may make the recommendation; grounds are similar to Section 5(2).

Sections 7 and 8 concern the application for, and description of powers of 'guardianship', intended to ensure that people over 16 years of age with an MD receive proper care and protection while living in the community. The guardian (who may be a relative) is nominated by the local authority and is empowered to ensure that the individual resides at a specified place, attends specified places and times for treatment, education, training or occupation and allows specified people (e.g. ASWs, doctors) access to their residence.

The Mental Health (Patients in the Community) Act 1995 came into force on 1 April 1996. This Act inserts new sections into the existing MHA 1983. The 1995 Act creates an entirely new legal status of 'After care under supervision (supervised discharge)'. An application for supervised discharge may be made only by the patient's RMO at a time when an individual is detained for treatment under the MHA 1983 under sections 3, 37, 47 or 48 and is an unrestricted patient. It is meant for people who need to be specifically supervised once they have left hospital to make sure they get the after-care they need. After-care may require the individual to live in a particular place; attend for medical treatment, occupation, education or training at set places and at set times. However, an individual cannot be forced to live at a certain place or take medication or any other kind of treatment without their consent while under supervised discharge. The patient and their NR both have the right to appeal to a MHRT when the application for supervised discharge is accepted, and every time it is reviewed.

Penal procedures and orders relating to prisoners

Section 35, empowering a Crown or Magistrates' Court to remand an accused person to a specific hospital for a report, lasts for 28 days, is applied for at trial by defence or prosecution council or by court and requires written or oral evidence from one medical practitioner.

Section 36, empowering a Crown Court to remand an accused individual to hospital for treatment is valid for 28 days and based on two medical reports (one from an 'approved doctor'); the person must be suffering from mental illness or severe mental impairment.

Section 37, empowers a Crown or Magistrates Court to order hospital admission or the reception into guardianship of a person convicted of an imprisonable offence (except murder).

Section 41, a restriction order (by Crown Court only) is based on the oral evidence of one doctor and added to hospital orders. Restricted patients may not be given leave, transferred or discharged without the consent of the Home Secretary.

Special issues

Section 57 concerns treatment requiring both consent *and* a second opinion (e.g. psychosurgery, surgical implants of hormones).

Section 58 concerns treatment requiring consent *or* a second opinion (e.g. electroconvulsive therapy [ECT], medications for longer than 6 months). This can be sought urgently.

Legislation for Scotland is different from the rest of the UK with new mental health and capacity acts already in place.

The Court of Protection is part of the Crown Court and provides for the protection and management of the property and affairs of persons incompetent to do so because of MD.

Risk assessment and management in psychiatry

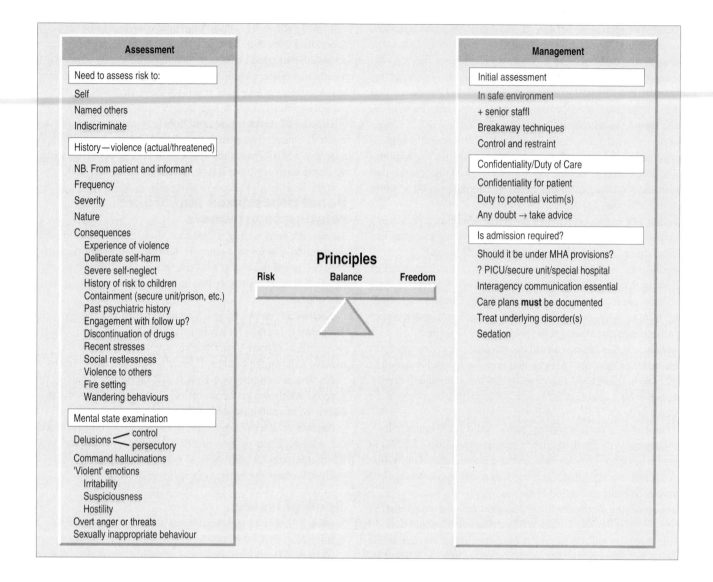

Assessment

Need to assess risk to:

Self

Named others

Indiscriminate

History—violence (actual/threatened)

NB. From patient and informant

Frequency

Severity

Nature

Consequences
- Experience of violence
- Deliberate self-harm
- Severe self-neglect
- History of risk to children
- Containment (secure unit/prison, etc.)
- Past psychiatric history
- Engagement with follow up?
- Discontinuation of drugs
- Recent stresses
- Social restlessness
- Violence to others
- Fire setting
- Wandering behaviours

Mental state examination

Delusions — control
         — persecutory

Command hallucinations

'Violent' emotions
- Irritability
- Suspiciousness
- Hostility

Overt anger or threats

Sexually inappropriate behaviour

Principles

Risk   Balance   Freedom

Management

Initial assessment

In safe environment

+ senior staffl

Breakaway techniques

Control and restraint

Confidentiality/Duty of Care

Confidentiality for patient

Duty to potential victim(s)

Any doubt → take advice

Is admission required?

Should it be under MHA provisions?

? PICU/secure unit/special hospital

Interagency communication essential

Care plans **must** be documented

Treat underlying disorder(s)

Sedation

One of the abiding principles in modern psychiatry is that patients' management should be as unrestrictive and normalizing as possible. Inevitably such an approach carries some degree of risk of harm to the patient or to others. There is thus a constant need to balance patients' rights and expectations against the resulting degree of risk. The aim of such risk assessment and management is to reduce risk as far as possible without undue restriction of individual freedoms. Risk cannot however be eliminated completely. Risks to be considered include those to the self, those specific to named others (e.g. in response to specific persecutory delusions or to a named person in a real or imagined vendetta) and those that are relatively indiscriminate, but are most likely to affect staff and other patients in the immediate vicinity.

Risk assessment

Risk assessment is mandatory when any patient with a psychiatric illness is admitted to hospital. Such assessment is also prudent in other contexts such as liaison and general practice psychiatry. Degree of risk is exquisitely sensitive both to changing circumstances and to a patient's changing mental state. Risk assessment should thus be a continuous process of monitoring both the patient and the care setting. The main factors to be considered in assessing the extent to which an individual patient currently poses a risk include aspects of the psychiatric history (including recent risk behaviours) and features within the current mental state.

Psychiatric history

Within the psychiatric history, one must note any history of violence (frequency, severity, nature and most serious harm resulting). A history of exposure to violence or abuse is also important. Any episodes of deliberate self-harm should be documented in detail (circumstances, method, management), as should any evidence of past severe self-neglect. One should also note any history of risk to children. Previous episodes of containment (compulsory detention, treatment in special hospital, secure unit, locked ward, prison or police station) are important and should be noted in detail where possible. Specific additional information within the psychiatric history should include extent of compliance with previous and current psychiatric treatment and after-care, alcohol or drug misuse (or any other disinhibiting factors) and extent of social integration. Past or current episodes of disengagement from psychiatric follow-up should be noted. Recent stressful life events or changes in life circumstances may be particularly important factors increasing current risk, as can recent discontinuation of prescribed or recreational drugs. More generally, evidence of 'social restlessness' such as frequent changes of relationships, work or domicile, indicate increased risk and should be documented.

Most of the above clinical features are indicators of increased risk of harm both to self and to others. Other factors predisposing to deliberate self-harm or actual suicide are discussed in detail in Chapter 7.

Several specific behaviour patterns are associated with increased risk to self or others and should be specifically enquired for in history taking from patient and informant as well as in perusal of case-notes and other documentation. These include episodes of accidental or deliberate harm to self or others, such as overdoses or deliberate self-injury; cigarette-burned bedclothes or deliberate fire-setting; wandering behaviours (particularly in the context of cognitive impairment); and falls consequent on alcohol or drug intoxication. Any such behaviour identified should be documented in detail as to timing, nature and severity of resultant harm.

Acts or threats of violence (to family, strangers, staff or other patients) should also be documented, as should any evidence of sexually inappropriate behaviour. Again, methods used and resultant injury should be noted. Risk to children or other vulnerable individuals (e.g. older people) should also be assessed. Both confidentiality (with regards the patient) and duty to the potential victim must be considered carefully and, if in doubt, advice taken from Trust lawyers, defence organizations, General Medical Council/British Medical Association or equivalent.

Initial assessment

Initial assessment of all patients, particularly those already identified as of high risk, should take place in as safe an environment as possible. The environment in which the patient is being examined or cared for should be assessed and modified to minimize risk. Potential patient access to harmful agents (firearms, knives, other weapons, incendiary devices) should be considered. Where risk is anticipated, one should ensure that senior staff are present where possible. Staff should be trained in 'breakaway' and where possible in 'control and restraint' techniques. Assessment areas should have appropriate alarm facilities and exit routes.

Within the mental state examination (see Chapter 1) key features in risk assessment include persecutory delusions (especially with specific person[s] involved), delusions of control or passivity phenomena, command hallucinations and emotions with a violent flavour (irritability, suspiciousness, hostility). Overt anger or explicit threats are particularly informative.

At the end of the initial assessment, it should be possible to estimate the level of risk in terms of seriousness, specificity, immediacy and potential for rapid change. This forms the basis of a management plan aimed at risk reduction.

Management

Clinical management of risk involves decisions as to whether admission is necessary, and if so whether such admission should be under the provisions of the Mental Health Act (MHA) (see Chapter 28) and/or to a psychiatric intensive care unit (PICU), secure unit or special hospital. Level of monitoring should be specified both for patients in the community and those in hospital. Medication may play an important role both in treating any underlying psychiatric disorder and also (in patients with high levels of arousal), in inducing sedation or tranquillization (see Chapters 33 and 34). Communication between agencies (particularly Health and Social Services) is crucial in planning future care in the community of patients at high risk who are likely to need considerable supervision that is both practical and acceptable. Care plans and their implementation must be negotiated by all involved parties (including patients themselves and their family and other informal carers) and fully documented.

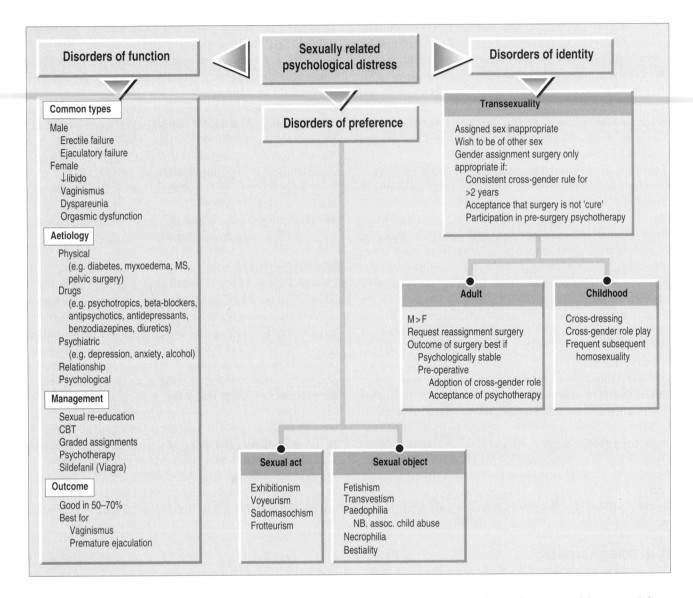

The range of sexual behaviour is extremely wide, with concepts of normality socially or legally, rather than physiologically, determined. Moral and legal objections to some forms of sexual behaviour and an increasing awareness of the potential hazards of sexual freedom (particularly human immunodeficiency virus [HIV] infection), and of what might be expected from a sexual relationship, have encouraged the increasing 'medicalization' of sexuality. Current psychiatric classifications (DSM-IV-TR, ICD-10) emphasize that sexual disorders have an element of psychological distress rather than being defined by behaviour alone. They can conveniently be divided into disorders of sexual *function*, *preference* and *identity*.

Sexual dysfunctions

Some degree of sexual dissatisfaction is present in as many as 20% of women and 30% of men. The commonest problems identified in both surveys and referrals to sexual disorder clinics are failure of erection and/or ejaculation in men; and low sexual interest, inability to allow penetration (vaginismus), pain on intercourse (dyspareunia), lack of sexual enjoyment and orgasmic dysfunction in women.

Assessment involves detailed history taking from, and examination of, both partners in order to identify the nature of the problem, its time course, the couple's knowledge of and attitudes to sex and the reasons why help is now being sought. Aetiological factors to be considered in the initial assessment include psychological factors, recent life events, specific medical and psychiatric conditions (and their treatment), past sexual abuse and poor general relationship with the sexual partner. Physical conditions impeding sexual function include neurological conditions (e.g. multiple sclerosis), diabetes, myxoedema and pelvic surgery. Sexual dysfunction may be induced by several drugs including beta-blockers, diuretics, antipsychotics (particularly thioridazine), benzodiazepines and most forms of antidepressant drugs. Sexual function is often impaired in depression (where loss of libido may reflect generalized anhedonia), alcohol dependence or abuse and anxiety states, and may be a manifestation of poor psychological adjustment to surgery (particularly mastectomy, colostomy or amputation).

Management increasingly involves a combination of medical and counselling interventions, including treatment of underlying medical or psychiatric conditions and couple therapy. Until recently erectile dysfunction in men was largely treated by physical means such as intracavernosal drugs such as prostaglandins or phentolamine, mechanical devices (vacuum pumps, penile bands), oral yohimbine or (rarely) surgical implants. Oral phosphodiesterase inhibitors such as sildefanil (Viagra) have largely superseded these interventions as the drug of choice for treatment for erectile dysfunction. Psychological treatments are essentially cognitive–behavioural, aiming at facilitating communication, decreasing anxiety about performance failure and identifying and exploring underlying psychodynamic problems as well as sexual re-education. This may include traditional sex therapy which (irrespective of the presenting dysfunction) involves the setting of a hierarchy of sexual 'assignments', structured on behavioural principles. Outcome is good in 50–70% of cases, the best results being for premature ejaculation in men and vaginismus in women. Other favourable prognostic factors include good quality of general relationship, high motivation and early progress within treatment.

Disorders of sexual preference

The paraphilias may be classified into those where the primary deviation is the focus for the sufferer's initial sexual arousal (rather than the subsequent sexual act) and those where it lies in the nature of the preferred sexual act itself.

It should be noted in this context that homosexuality is not considered a disorder of sexual preference. Subjects who are dissatisfied with their sexual orientation are almost always so because of prejudice or discrimination.

Variations of the sexual object include *paedophilia* (sexual activity or fantasy involving children); *fetishism* (where the object of sexual arousal is an inanimate object [e.g. an item of clothing or a non-genital body part]); *transvestism* (where sexual arousal is obtained by cross-dressing); and, more rarely, *bestiality* (sexual activity with animals) and *necrophilia* (intercourse with a dead body). Paedophilia is particularly important because of its link with child pornography and abuse (see Chapter 21). The aetiology of these conditions is unclear; management usually involves behaviour therapy (which may involve elements both of aversion and of conditioning more appropriate responses). Antiandrogens are sometimes used in paedophilia.

Variations of the sexual act involve the induction of both sexual arousal and (usually) orgasm by specific actions. Almost all people presenting to the courts or for psychiatric treatment with such variations are men. The commonest form is *exhibitionism* (indecent exposure) in which genital exposure is accompanied by emotional tension and excitement as well as sexual arousal. Exhibitionists make up one-quarter of the sexual offences dealt with by the courts, with psychiatric referral usually by this route. Exhibitionists fall into two main groups: those with aggressive personality traits or even antisocial personality disorders (see Chapter 12) and in whom the act frequently involves masturbation; and those of inhibited temperament, where the exposed penis is often flaccid. Treatment may include psychodynamic, behavioural and hormonal (antiandrogen) components.

Other relatively common variations of the sexual act include *voyeurism* (observing sexual acts), *frotteurism* (rubbing the genitalia against a stranger in a crowded place) and *sadomasochism* (inflicting pain on others [sadism] or having it inflicted on oneself [masochism]). There are no systematic trials of treatment, although behavioural techniques are often used.

Disorders of sexual identity (DSI)

This involves a strong wish to be of the other sex, and a conviction that one's assigned sex is inappropriate. It may occur in children, in whom it is characterized by cross-dressing, taking cross-gender roles in games and fantasy and an attraction for pastimes appropriate to the other gender's stereotype. Whereas boys who show gender atypical behaviour often grow up to be gay, boys with clinical DSI do not regard themselves as gay as they grow up but rather as a woman (in a man's body) who is attracted to men.

The cardinal feature of DSI in adults (*transsexuality*) is a clear wish to live as a member of the other sex, with cross-dressing reflecting this rather than for sexual excitement. Most adult transsexuals are men. Transsexuals usually seek gender-reassignment surgery (with associated hormonal treatment). Outcome following such treatment is best where the patient is otherwise psychologically stable, has adopted the cross-gender role consistently for at least 2 years prior to surgery, accepts that surgical treatment is not a 'cure' and is willing to participate in presurgical psychotherapy.

31 Psychiatric aspects of HIV and AIDS

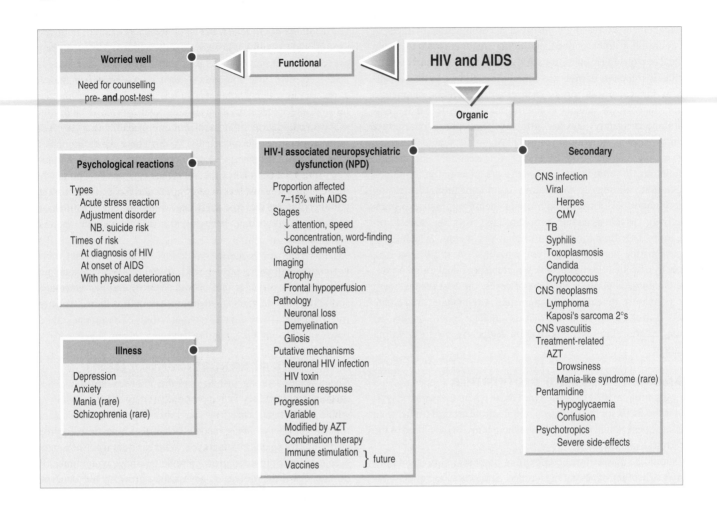

The World Health Organization estimated that at the end of 2004, 39.4 million people were living with human immunodeficiency virus (HIV) or acquired immunodeficiency syndrome (AIDS) and a further 20 million had died of AIDS-related illnesses. In the developed world the majority of cases were, until recently, in homosexual men and in intravenous drug abusers, but the incidence of heterosexually spread HIV infection is rising rapidly, particularly in adolescents and in women. Associated psychological problems range from fear of infection in the 'worried well', through psychological reactions to being HIV infected or developing features of AIDS, to functional psychiatric disorders in those with established HIV or full-blown AIDS and neuropsychiatric syndromes resulting both from HIV itself and from its complications and treatment.

The worried well

People (not all of whom are at risk of HIV) may become preoccupied with the possibility of becoming infected; this may present with repeated requests for HIV serological testing. HIV testing should never be undertaken without clarification of why the test is being sought, estimation of likelihood of a positive result and advice as to further action whatever the test result. It also provides an opportunity for education on minimizing high-risk behaviour. A request for testing may reflect underlying depression or anxiety, which should be excluded or treated as part of the initial assessment. More rarely, patients with psychotic depression or schizophrenia may present with the delusion that they are HIV positive.

Psychological reactions to HIV infection

Patients with HIV may undergo periods of crisis on first learning that they are infected, when they first develop an HIV-related illness or full-blown AIDS and as physical deterioration becomes inexorable. They may react to these crises with acute stress reactions or more insidious adjustment reactions (see Chapter 8). Risk of deliberate self-harm must be considered. This is particularly important in the context of disclosure of a positive HIV-test. Such disclosure should be prearranged and in person; where possible a close friend or family member should be present, and one or more follow-up appointments may be needed. Patients may initially display shock or disavowal; they should be encouraged to ventilate their feelings and supported through the anger and despair that often precede acceptance of the diagnosis. Self-help groups can play an important role.

Functional psychiatric disorders

Depressive symptoms are common at all stages of HIV and AIDS. The diagnosis of depressive illness may be difficult. Low mood may be an understandable reaction to the diagnosis or to progressive disability, and apathy due to organic central nervous system (CNS) disease. Anhedonia, hopelessness and suicidal thinking are, however, likely to reflect true depressive illness and warrant treatment. HIV-positive patients may also present with acute mania or schizophrenia-like psychoses. Anxiety is also common, and may respond to behavioural and/or pharmacological treatment. Organic aetiology should be excluded or treated; the principles of management of functional psychoses are not altered by comorbidity with HIV or AIDS.

People with AIDS are often very sensitive to the side-effects of psychotropic drugs. The anticholinergic effects of tricyclic antidepressants can aggravate cognitive deficits, and selective serotonin reuptake inhibitors (SSRIs) may be preferred. Similarly, benzodiazepines and antipsychotics may also aggravate organic presentations. Choice of psychotropic is often dictated by the patient's physical problems. For example, where depression coexists with the chronic diarrhoea common in AIDS, patients may benefit from the anticholinergic effects of tricyclics but be intolerant of SSRIs.

HIV-induced neuropsychiatric dysfunction (NPD)

Some subjects infected with HIV (estimates vary between 10% and 90%) develop self-limiting aseptic meningitis, which probably represents the entry of the virus into the CNS. The clinical presentation is usually of a glandular fever-like illness accompanied by neck stiffness, but there may also be a transient confusional state.

Later in the disease, HIV-positive subjects may develop persistent and progressive cognitive changes. These are thought to be a direct manifestation of HIV infection within the brain and are known as HIV-I associated dementia (NPD). NPD develops rarely in patients with AIDS-related complex, and in about 7–15% of those with untreated AIDS.

The early stages of NPD may be apparent only on detailed neuropsychological testing, particularly on measures of psychomotor speed or of sustained attention. Rarely, however, there may be a more acute presentation with a mania-like agitated psychosis accompanied by acute impairment of memory and orientation.

As NPD develops, the picture is of a subcortical dementia in which difficulties become apparent in concentration, word-finding, memory and information processing. The cognitive changes may be accompanied by apathy, social withdrawal and motor dysfunction (hand tremor, deteriorating handwriting, poor balance). The later stages of NPD are characterized by a clinical picture similar to that of other dementias, with progressive impairment of daily living skills leading to inability to converse and full physical dependency.

Structural imaging scans in NPD reveal cortical atrophy (which may precede cognitive impairments) and, less frequently, patchy areas of low attenuation in the white matter. Single photo emission tomography (SPECT) studies reveal frontal hypoperfusion. The main pathological abnormalities are demyelination and gliosis, more marked in white matter, and grey-matter neuronal loss. Postulated pathogenic mechanisms include direct infection of neurons and glia by HIV, toxin production and host immune responses.

The prognosis of NPD is variable and treatment dependent. Before azidothymidine (AZT) came into routine use in the treatment of AIDS, some patients with NPD showed very rapid cognitive deterioration over weeks. AZT may temporarily reverse or delay progression of the cognitive deficits of early NPD, and subsequent cognitive decline can take 1 year or more. There is early evidence that newer combination antiviral therapies can slow or reverse NPD, though their efficiencies vary. It is possible that in the future combination therapies, immune stimulation and/or selective vaccines may prevent NPD. There are currently no other specific treatments for NPD. Agitation may require antipsychotics, although NPD renders patients particularly vulnerable to severe and prolonged extrapyramidal side-effects. Psychostimulants such as methylphenidate may transiently improve both mood and cognitive performance.

Neuropsychiatric manifestations of complications of HIV

Severely immunocompromised AIDS patients are vulnerable to a variety of opportunistic CNS infections. Viral infections include herpes and cytomegalovirus (CMV). Non-viral infections are also common. These include tuberculosis (TB), syphilis, toxoplasmosis, candidiasis and cryptococcal meningitis. AIDS also renders patients vulnerable to CNS neoplasia, particularly lymphoma (primary or secondary) and metastatic Kaposi's sarcoma. CNS vasculitis can result in haemorrhage or infarction. These complications may present with non-specific cognitive deterioration or more florid acute confusional states, with or without focal neurological signs.

Treatments directed at HIV and its complications can also result in neuropsychiatric syndromes. AZT can cause drowsiness or, rarely, a mania-like syndrome. Pentamidine (used in the treatment and prophylaxis of cryptococcal lung infections) may induce hypoglycaemia and resultant confusion.

Type	Frequency	Number of sessions	Key principles/contents	Main indications
Psychoanalysis	3–5/week	Hundreds	Unconscious defence mechanisms Transference	Personality disorders Psychosexual difficulties Psychosomatic problems
BPP	1–2/week	Variable	Psychological conflicts underlying interpersonal problems	Personality disorders Psychosexual difficulties Psychosomatic problems
IPT	Weekly	12–16	Detailed interpersonal inventory Focus on 1 of Role transitions Role disputes Grief and loss Social anxiety	Depression (non-psychotic) Eating disorders
CBT	Weekly	6–12	Negative cognitions Self World Future	Depression Anxiety Eating disorders Schizophrenia Some personality disorders
BT	Weekly	6–12	Learning theory Desensitization Operant conditioning Activity schedules	Depression Pain management Recovery after coma or myocardial infarction
DBT	Weekly or more frequent	Variable	Dialectical dilemmas Hierarchy of targets	Borderline personality disorder
Counselling	Weekly	Variable	Wide range of interventions including Person-centred Non-directive Problem-solving Supportive	Primary care and medical settings

Psychotherapy (based on verbal communication between client/patient [CP] and doctor, and the relationship between them) aims to help individual CPs cope, adjust to life, relieve uncomfortable psychological symptoms, improve their mental state and/or foster their rehabilitation. Psychotherapeutic approaches form an important part of general clinical management. More specific therapies may be categorized into psychoanalysis, brief effective therapies and supportive therapies.

Psychoanalysis

Psychoanalysis stems from the school of psychology founded by Sigmund Freud. Despite considerable modification, the central notion remains that human behaviour is determined predominantly by unconscious forces derived from primitive emotional needs, rather than by reason. Therapy aims to resolve long-standing underlying conflicts and unconscious defence mechanisms (e.g. denial, repression), to promote personal growth and modify the CP's personality by exploring the unconscious using free-association (the CP saying whatever enters his/her mind) and interpretation. An analyst sees a CP four or five times a week for 50–60 minutes for 2–5 years. One key therapeutic tool is the 'transference' (whereby the CP transfers to the analyst strong emotions experienced in early important relationships). 'Counter-transference' refers to thoughts and feelings the analyst experiences towards the CP. Psychoanalytic concepts provide a historical context and concepts relevant to the more focused psychotherapies (see below).

Brief effective therapies
Brief psychodynamic psychotherapy (BPP)

BPP is related to but more widely available than psychoanalysis. It aims to facilitate changes by detecting and resolving underlying psychological conflicts which cause interpersonal problems. Treatment sessions are less frequent (one to two times a week).

Interpersonal psychotherapy (IPT)

IPT arises from research linking interpersonal relationships, life events and social networks with depression (see Chapter 5). It is in wide use in the USA. A detailed interpersonal inventory is taken of all close relationships. A particular focus is chosen such as role transitions (e.g. promotion, loss of job, becoming a parent) or disputes within important relationships. Other foci include grief and social anxiety. Fluctuations in the area of focus are carefully matched to fluctuating symptoms on the basis that if the interpersonal difficulty can be helped the underlying depression will be alleviated. IPT has also been used successfully in eating disorders.

Cognitive–behaviour therapy (CBT)

CBT is based on observations that depressed patients entertain negatively biased cognitions (thoughts) of themselves, their future and the environment/world (Beck's cognitive triad). These cognitive distortions (or processing errors) maintain people's negative convictions in the face of contrary evidence. They are thought to arise from early traumatic experiences and, in depression, are manifest as 'automatic thoughts' which the CP is encouraged to challenge. CBT seeks to change these important inner attitudes. CBT is also used in the treatment of anxiety, eating disorders, schizophrenia and some personality disorders.

Behaviour therapy (BT)

BT, based on learning theory, concentrates on changing behaviour. Techniques include exposure, response prevention, habituation and thought stopping. Operant conditioning involves encouraging desirable behaviours by positive reinforcement, and discouraging undesirable behaviours by withholding reinforcement (extinction). In aversion therapy, now seldom used, the CP is given an unpleasant stimulus when behaviour is undesirable. In 'flooding', the CP is rapidly exposed to a real or imagined anxiety-producing stimulus. In systematic desensitization (SD) the CP experiences graded exposure to a hierarchy of anxiety producing situations. Reciprocal inhibition couples SD with a response incompatible with anxiety (e.g. relaxation, eating). BT has recently shifted towards using activity schedules, reducing avoidance and self-monitoring, backed by education and information. Such regimes are effective in depression, recovery after coma or myocardial infarction and pain management.

Habit reversal training (HRT) has been shown to be superior to supportive psychotherapy in Tourette syndrome.

Dialectical behaviour therapy (DBT)

DBT, an empirically validated treatment specifically designed for individuals with borderline personality disorder (BPD), is based on a theoretical model in which the central problem in BPD is 'self-invalidation' resulting from a set of 'dialectical dilemmas'. The goal of therapy is to achieve a balance or 'synthesis'. Therapy also involves invoking and resolving dialectical opposites (e.g. acceptance/change; experiencing/reducing emotions) and is structured in stages. At each stage a defined hierarchy of targets is defined.

Group therapy emphases interrelationships within the group where problems are shared. Groups (12 members are ideal) meet weekly, and run for months to years. The therapist adopts a non-directive role but discourages CPs from avoiding 'psychological work' (e.g. remaining silent or invoking irrelevancies).

Family therapy (FT) may be *systemic* or *behavioural*. Systemic FT has a central premise that problems have arisen with the system of family functioning rather than with just the individual. It is used predominantly in child and adolescent psychiatry. The expectation is that improved family functioning will result in improvement in the index 'case'. Behavioural FT follows similar principles to individual behaviour therapy and is largely used for severe mental disorders.

Milieu therapy, within an in-patient 'Therapeutic Community', employs all residents (CPs) and staff to give support to individual CPs, promoting adaptive coping skills and appropriate behaviour by peer pressure.

Transactional analysis (TA) was founded by Eric Berne who noted that individuals related to each other in different ego states (children, adults, parents). In TA these ego states are explored/interpreted to the CP (individually or in groups), aiming at predominantly adult functioning.

Supportive therapies
Counselling

The term covers a wide range of different and largely unproven interventions. The most widely practiced is person-centred counselling. This is non-directive; the aim is to 'be with' the CP in a meaningful way. Empathy, unconditional positivity and genuineness are the main therapeutic ingredients. Other types of counselling involving provision of information, problem solving and support have been shown to be effective in primary care and general medical settings.

Supportive psychotherapy (SP)

SP, the simplest form of psychotherapy, assesses the CP's life situation by allowing the CP to talk freely about his/herself, symptoms and problems. CPs are seen weekly for several weeks or months. Brief (one to three sessions) crisis intervention helps support an individual at times of stress or crisis and prevent breakdown of functioning. The therapist works with the CP's symptoms rather than unconscious processes, and does not aim at major personality changes or giving insight. He/she listens to the CP, understands the problems and reinforces psychological defence mechanisms. Cooperation from the CP (trying to solve problems, rather than dependence and regression) is stressed. Suggested steps are establishing rapport, facilitating the expression of affect/emotions (e.g. grief, anger), followed by reflection, clarification, reassurance from the therapist, facilitation of the CP's understanding of his/her own feelings and encouragement of problem-solving behaviour.

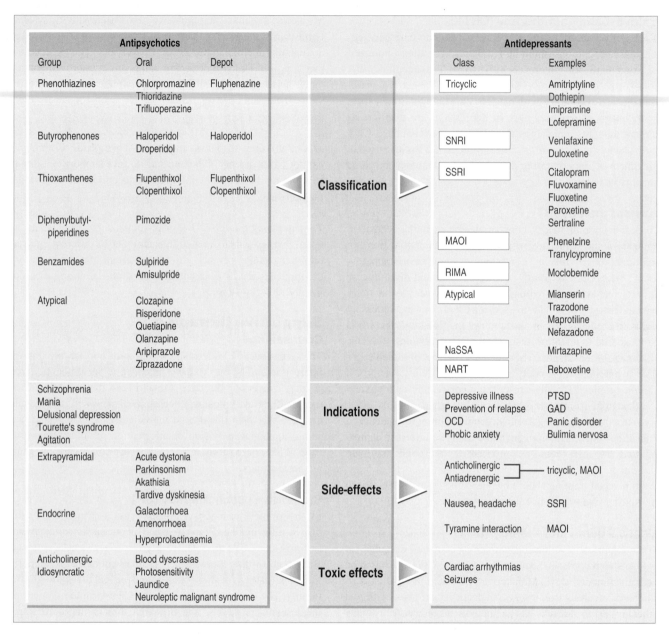

Antipsychotics		
Group	Oral	Depot
Phenothiazines	Chlorpromazine	Fluphenazine
	Thioridazine	
	Trifluoperazine	
Butyrophenones	Haloperidol	Haloperidol
	Droperidol	
Thioxanthenes	Flupenthixol	Flupenthixol
	Clopenthixol	Clopenthixol
Diphenylbutyl-piperidines	Pimozide	
Benzamides	Sulpiride	
	Amisulpride	
Atypical	Clozapine	
	Risperidone	
	Quetiapine	
	Olanzapine	
	Aripiprazole	
	Ziprazadone	

Classification

Antidepressants	
Class	Examples
Tricyclic	Amitriptyline
	Dothiepin
	Imipramine
	Lofepramine
SNRI	Venlafaxine
	Duloxetine
SSRI	Citalopram
	Fluvoxamine
	Fluoxetine
	Paroxetine
	Sertraline
MAOI	Phenelzine
	Tranylcypromine
RIMA	Moclobemide
Atypical	Mianserin
	Trazodone
	Maprotiline
	Nefazadone
NaSSA	Mirtazapine
NART	Reboxetine

Indications

Schizophrenia	
Mania	
Delusional depression	
Tourette's syndrome	
Agitation	

Depressive illness	PTSD
Prevention of relapse	GAD
OCD	Panic disorder
Phobic anxiety	Bulimia nervosa

Side-effects

Extrapyramidal	Acute dystonia
	Parkinsonism
	Akathisia
	Tardive dyskinesia
Endocrine	Galactorrhoea
	Amenorrhoea
	Hyperprolactinaemia

Anticholinergic / Antiadrenergic	tricyclic, MAOI
Nausea, headache	SSRI
Tyramine interaction	MAOI

Toxic effects

Anticholinergic	Blood dyscrasias
Idiosyncratic	Photosensitivity
	Jaundice
	Neuroleptic malignant syndrome

Cardiac arrhythmias
Seizures

Physical treatments should always be seen as part of individual patients' management programmes rather than as complete in themselves. There is also no intrinsic antagonism between physical and more social or psychological treatment approaches; indeed, they are usually complementary.

Antipsychotics

The first, chlorpromazine, was introduced in 1951 for use in anaesthetic premedication since it induced a state of 'relaxed alertness'. It was soon tried in schizophrenia and noted to reduce delusions and hallucinations without causing excessive sedation.

Drugs currently in use are the phenothiazines (such as chlorpromazine, thioridazine, fluphenazine and trifluoperazine); the butyrophenones (haloperidol, droperidol); the thioxanthenes (flupenthixol, *cis*-clopenthixol); the diphenylbutylpiperidines (pimozide) and the substituted benzamides (sulpiride, amisulpride); and the atypical antipsychotics clozapine, olanzapine, quetiapine, risperidone, ziprasidone and aripiprazole. The latter two are newest on the market and both are thought to act primarily through $5HT_{2A}$ antagonism.

Mechanism of action. All antipsychotics are potent dopamine-receptor blockers but also block cholinergic, adrenergic and histaminic receptors. Older drugs (phenothiazines and butyrophenones) are relatively non-selective, whereas the benzamides are highly selective blockers of D2 dopamine receptors. The 'atypical' antipsychotics block $5HT_2$ receptors as well as dopamine receptors. Some atypicals preferentially block limbic dopamine receptors in the striatum.

Mode of administration. This is usually by mouth, with extensive 'first-pass' metabolism in the liver. Many can also be given by short-acting intramuscular (IM) or intravenous (IV) injection. Some (such as haloperidol, flupenthixol and risperidone) can be given by 'depot' injection every 1–4 weeks. This bypasses first-pass metabolism and may improve compliance. Depot medication is easier to monitor. The supervising community nurse can also act as the 'care co-ordinator'.

Indications. Antipsychotics are drugs of first choice in the treatment of schizophrenia; they are most effective in alleviating 'positive' symptoms such as delusions, hallucinations, disorders of possession of thought and formal thought disorder; they are also effective in preventing relapse. Clozapine and risperidone may be more effective against 'negative' features (lack of volition and poverty of thought and affect) than other neuroleptics. Antipsychotics are also effective in the treatment of mania and Tourette's syndrome. They are also used, in combination with antidepressants, in delusional depression. Atypical antipsychotics are no longer much used for violent or agitated behaviour in older people because of concerns about increased risk of stroke and impairment of glycaemic control.

Side-effects. The most important of these are the extrapyramidal movement disorders. Patients may experience acute dystonic reactions (torticollis, oculogyric crisis, increased muscle tone), parkinsonism or akathisia (psychomotor restlessness). Acute dystonia and parkinsonism reflect drug-induced dopamine/acetylchoine imbalance and respond to anticholinergic drugs such as procyclidine. Akathisia is less responsive to anticholinergics than parkinsonism. Beta-blockers or benzodiazepines may be helpful. Long-term antipsychotics may cause tardive dyskinesia (TD), thought to be due to dopamine-receptor supersensitivity and characterized by abnormal buccolingual masticatory movements and, in severe cases, choreiform trunk and limb movements, especially in older people. Tetrabenazine may reduce the movements of TD as may reduction or cessation of antipsychotics. TD is, however, irreversible in 50% of cases. Weight gain is an important and distressing side-effect associated with chronic antipsychotic administration and may adversely effect compliance. Most other side-effects relate to other receptor blockade. Anticholinergic effects include dry mouth, confusion and urinary retention. Postural hypotension and impotence are antiadrenergic effects and sedation probably reflects histamine blockade. Endocrine effects (secondary to dopamine blockade) include hyperprolactinaemia, amenorrhoea and galactorrhoea. Clozapine may cause potentially fatal agranulocytosis and seizures. Despite these risks and the need for regular haematological monitoring, clozapine is increasingly seen as useful in patients unresponsive to or intolerant of standard antipsychotics.

Toxic effects include the neuroleptic malignant syndrome (hyperpyrexia, autonomic instability, confusion and increased muscle tone); and (with phenothiazines) blood dyscrasias, retinal pigmentation, photosensitivity and cholestatic jaundice.

Antidepressants

Drugs currently in use may be divided into the tricyclics (such as imipramine, amitriptyline, dothiepin and lofepramine); the monoamine oxidase inhibitors (MAOIs) such as phenelzine and tranylcypromine and the new reversible inhibitor of MAO-A, or 'RIMA' moclobemide; the selective serotonin reuptake inhibitors (SSRIs) (citalopram, fluvoxamine, fluoxetine, sertraline and paroxetine); venlafaxine and duloxetine, selective serotonin and noradrenaline reuptake inhibitors [SNRIs]); mirtazapine, which has a noradrenergic and selective serotonergic action (NaSSA); the noradrenaline-selective reuptake inhibitor (NARI) reboxetine; and the atypical antidepressants including trazodone, maprotiline, mianserin and nefazodone. The herbal preparation hypericum (St John's Wort), whose active ingredient is thought to be hypericin, is widely used and may be effective in mild to moderate depression. Its action is similar to that of MAOIs and it may interact adversely with many other drugs.

Mechanism of action. Tricylics and SNRIs block reuptake of both noradrenaline and serotonin into the presynaptic neurone; SSRIs have a similar action on serotonin alone. MAOIs inhibit the breakdown of serotonin (and to a lesser extent noradrenaline) at the synapse. Mianserin and mirtazapine block presynaptic α_2-receptors. Any common mechanism of action for antidepressants probably involves modulation of pre- and/or post-synaptic receptors or electrophysiological responses.

Mode of administration. This is by mouth. Most antidepressants can be given once daily and are extensively and variably metabolized by first pass in the liver. The antidepressant response seldom occurs in less than 2 weeks and may not be fully apparent for 6 weeks, though early partial response is predictive of remission. Patients not warned of the delayed therapeutic action are likely to be poorly compliant.

Indications. The main indication for antidepressants is depressive illness. Patients with biological features of depression but no delusions are likeliest to respond; moderate to severe 'neurotic' depressions may also benefit. Studies suggest a response rate of 60–70% (compared to 30% with placebo). Antidepressants are also useful in phobic anxiety, panic disorder, bulimia nervosa, post-traumatic stress disorder (PTSD), general anxiety disorder (GAD), obsessive–compulsive disorder (OCD) (NB. higher doses may be needed) and in preventing depressive relapse.

Side-effects. Include anticholinergic and antiadrenergic effects similar to those of the antipsychotics. In overdose they may trigger potentially fatal cardiac arrhythmias and seizures. Lofepramine is relatively safe in overdose and free of anticholinergic effects. SSRIs are largely devoid of tricyclic-like side-effects but may cause headache, anorexia and nausea and occasional hyponatraemia, especially in older patients. There is increasing recent awareness that SSRIs and SNRIs may increase agitation during the first 1–2 weeks of use, and may also be associated with dysphoria and a range of unpleasant withdrawal phenomena if stopped abruptly. Gradual tapering over 2–4 weeks is recommended. MAOIs (not moclobemide) can cause an occasionally fatal syndrome of hypertension and throbbing headache if foods containing large quantities of tyramine (e.g. cheese, red wine) are eaten.

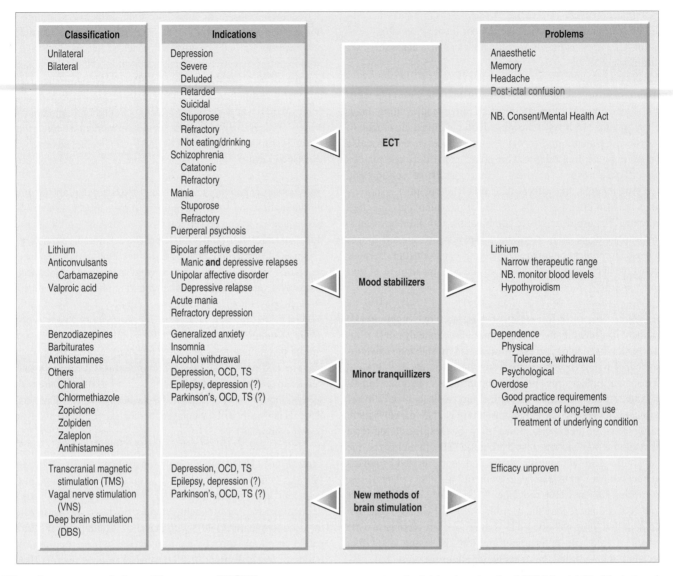

Classification	Indications		Problems

Unilateral
Bilateral
	Depression
	  Severe
	  Deluded
	  Retarded
	  Suicidal
	  Stuporose
	  Refractory
	  Not eating/drinking
	Schizophrenia
	  Catatonic
	  Refractory
	Mania
	  Stuporose
	  Refractory
	Puerperal psychosis
		ECT	Anaesthetic
			Memory
			Headache
			Post-ictal confusion
			
			NB. Consent/Mental Health Act

Lithium
Anticonvulsants
  Carbamazepine
Valproic acid
	Bipolar affective disorder
	  Manic **and** depressive relapses
	Unipolar affective disorder
	  Depressive relapse
	Acute mania
	Refractory depression
		Mood stabilizers	Lithium
			  Narrow therapeutic range
			  NB. monitor blood levels
			  Hypothyroidism

Benzodiazepines
Barbiturates
Antihistamines
Others
  Chloral
  Chlormethiazole
  Zopiclone
  Zolpiden
  Zaleplon
  Antihistamines
	Generalized anxiety
	Insomnia
	Alcohol withdrawal
	Depression, OCD, TS
	Epilepsy, depression (?)
	Parkinson's, OCD, TS (?)
		Minor tranquillizers	Dependence
			  Physical
			    Tolerance, withdrawal
			  Psychological
			Overdose
			  Good practice requirements
			    Avoidance of long-term use
			    Treatment of underlying condition

Transcranial magnetic
  stimulation (TMS)
Vagal nerve stimulation
  (VNS)
Deep brain stimulation
  (DBS)
	Depression, OCD, TS
	Epilepsy, depression (?)
	Parkinson's, OCD, TS (?)
		New methods of
		brain stimulation
			Efficacy unproven

Electroconvulsive therapy (ECT)

Mechanism of action

ECT involves the induction of a modified epileptic seizure. A series of such treatments induces complex effects including neurotransmitter release; a transient increase in blood–brain barrier permeability; secretion of hypothalamic and pituitary hormones; and modulation of neurotransmitter receptors similar to those induced by antidepressant drugs.

Mode of administration

ECT is given two or three times a week, usually to a total of between four and 12 treatments. Before each treatment the patient is fasted for at least 4 hours and is then given a short-acting anaesthetic, a muscle relaxant drug and a few seconds preoxygenation prior to the application of an electric current sufficient to trigger an epileptic seizure. This is given through electrodes placed bitemporally or with both on the non-dominant hemisphere. In England and Wales, ECT can only be given if *either* the patient has given informed consent *or* is detained under the 1983 Mental Health Act and an independent consultant appointed by the Mental Health Act Commissioners agrees that ECT must be given. In the latter situation, ECT can be initiated prior to the independent consultant's assessment under the provisions of Section 62 of the Mental Health Act.

Indications

The main indication for ECT is severe depression. Patients with depressive delusions and/or psychomotor retardation are likeliest to respond. Response rates may be as high as 90%. ECT should also be considered in depressed patients at high risk of suicide or not eating and drinking; those in whom other treatments have failed; in catatonic schizophrenia; in puerperal psychoses; and in otherwise unresponsive schizophrenia or mania. Speed of response may be faster than that of antidepressants.

Contraindications

There are no absolute contraindications to ECT. Raised intracranial pressure, recent stroke, recent myocardial infarction and crescendo angina are important relative contraindications.

Side-effects

Side-effects include anaesthetic complications, dysrhythmias due to vagal stimulation, post-ictal headache and confusion and retro- and anterograde amnesia with difficulties in registration and recall that may persist for several weeks. Memory problems are reduced by unilateral electrode placement which may, however, be slightly less effective.

New methods of brain stimulation

Transcranial magnetic stimulation (TMS; the prefrontal cortex is stimulated by the application of a strong magnetic field) has shown promise in the treatment of depression, OCD and Tourette's Syndrome (TS). Vagal nerve stimulation (VNS) is used in epilepsy and has antidepressant effects. In deep brain stimulation (DBS) a thin electrode is inserted directly into the brain and currents applied. It has been used in Parkinson's disease, OCD and TS. None of these techniques is yet establishd in clinical practice outside the USA.

Mood stabilizers

The most important of these is lithium (discussed below); carbamazepine (which may be particularly useful in rapid-cycling bipolar illness), valproic acid and lamotrigine are also used. There is some evidence for the efficacy of calcium channel blockers such as nifedipine.

Indications

The main indications for lithium are prophylaxis in recurrent affective disorder (unipolar and bipolar), acute treatment of mania and augmentation of antidepressants in resistant depression. Lithium may also be used in schizoaffective illness and in the control of aggression.

Mode of administration

Lithium is taken by mouth and excreted by the kidneys. It has a narrow therapeutic range (0.5–1.5 mmol/L). Prior to lithium therapy, thyroid and renal function should be evaluated. Serum lithium levels should be monitored regularly (initially weekly, thereafter every 12 weeks), blood being taken 8–12 hours after last dose. In patients on lithium, renal and thyroid function tests and in those on carbamazepine, full blood count (FBC) should be monitored every 6 months. Patients should be warned that an unexplained sore throat may herald agranulocytosis.

Mechanism of action

Lithium interacts with all biological systems where sodium, potassium, calcium or magnesium are involved. At therapeutic blood levels it probably has effects on neurotransmission including 5HT, noradrenaline, dopamine and acetylchlorine. Its interference with cyclic adenosine monophosphate (cAMP)-linked receptors explains its action on the thyroid and kidney.

Side-effects and toxic effects

Side-effects of lithium include nausea, fine tremor, weight gain, oedema, polydipsia, polyuria, exacerbation of psoriasis and acne and hypothyroidism. Toxicity is indicated by vomiting, diarrhoea, coarse tremor, slurred speech, ataxia, drowsiness, confusion, convulsions and coma. Treatment of toxicity/overdose involves cessation of lithium, forced diuresis (intravenous mannitol), haemodialysis or peritoneal dialysis. Carbamazepine may cause blood dyscrasias and rashes.

Contraindications

Lithium should be avoided in renal, cardiac, thyroid and Addison's disease and in pregnancy and breastfeeding. Dehydration and diuretics can lead to lithium toxicity. Adverse interactions can also occur between lithium and non-steroidal anti-inflammatory drugs, calcium channel blockers and some antibiotics. Carbamazepine is also teratogenic and may interfere with the action of oral contraceptives, necessitating other contraceptive precautions.

Minor tranquillizers

The most important of these are the benzodiazepines (BDZs); these were preceded by the barbiturates and chloral hydrate.

Drugs currently in use and indications

As the BDZs are anxiolytic, sleep inducing, anticonvulsant and muscle relaxants, their indications include insomnia, generalized (but not phobic) anxiety, alcohol withdrawal states and the control of violent behaviour. Underlying conditions (such as depression) should always be excluded and behavioural alternative treatments considered. BDZs are also used as 'second-line' drugs in refractory epilepsy. Chlormethiazole, zopiclone, zolpiden, zaleplon and antihistamines such as promethazine may be used as hypnotics. Buspirone has anxiolytic effects.

Mode of administration

The main mode of administration is oral, but intramuscular, intravenous or rectal administration may be required in status epilepticus and in violent patients.

Pharmacokinetics

Most have active metabolites, some with half-lives of several days. The long-acting BDZs include diazepam, chlordiazepoxide and nitrazepam; lorazepam, oxazepam and temazepam are shorter-acting BDZs.

Mechanism of action

Mechanism of action of BDZs and most other minor tranquillizers (apart from antihistamines) is potentiation of the inhibitory effects of γ-aminobutyric acid (GABA).

Toxic and side-effects

Toxic effects and side-effects of minor tranquillizers include drowsiness, sedation, ataxia, respiratory depression and disinhibition which may lead (paradoxically) to aggression. Tolerance to BDZs frequently occurs, and there is a prolonged withdrawal syndrome, with marked anxiety, shakiness, abdominal cramps, perceptual disturbances, persecutory delusions and fits. They should therefore usually only be prescribed for no more than a couple of weeks. Weaning patients off BDZs to which they have (iatrogenically) become dependent may take months or even years.

Contraindications

BDZs potentiate alcohol and other minor tranquillizers; the combination is dangerous in overdose.

35 Cross-cultural psychiatry

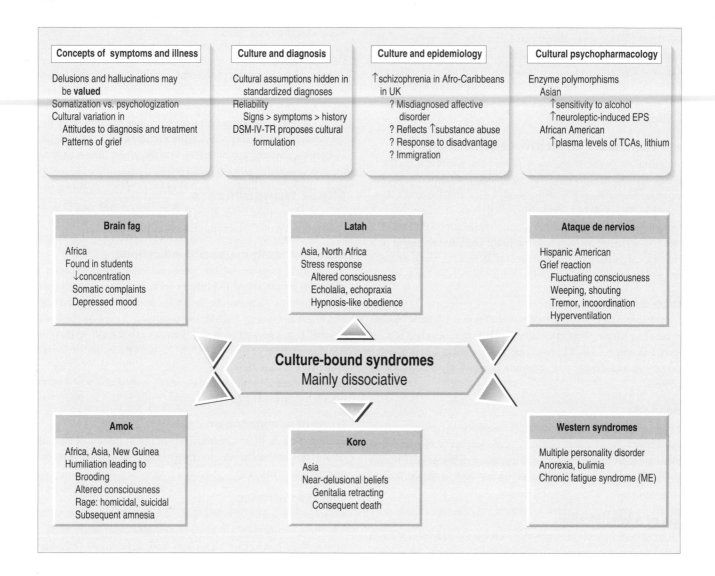

Concepts of symptoms and illness

Delusions and hallucinations may be **valued**
Somatization vs. psychologization
Cultural variation in
 Attitudes to diagnosis and treatment
 Patterns of grief

Culture and diagnosis

Cultural assumptions hidden in standardized diagnoses
Reliability
 Signs > symptoms > history
DSM-IV-TR proposes cultural formulation

Culture and epidemiology

↑schizophrenia in Afro-Caribbeans in UK
 ? Misdiagnosed affective disorder
 ? Reflects ↑substance abuse
 ? Response to disadvantage
 ? Immigration

Cultural psychopharmacology

Enzyme polymorphisms
Asian
 ↑sensitivity to alcohol
 ↑neuroleptic-induced EPS
African American
 ↑plasma levels of TCAs, lithium

Brain fag

Africa
Found in students
 ↓concentration
 Somatic complaints
 Depressed mood

Latah

Asia, North Africa
Stress response
 Altered consciousness
 Echolalia, echopraxia
 Hypnosis-like obedience

Ataque de nervios

Hispanic American
Grief reaction
 Fluctuating consciousness
 Weeping, shouting
 Tremor, incoordination
 Hyperventilation

Culture-bound syndromes
Mainly dissociative

Amok

Africa, Asia, New Guinea
Humiliation leading to
 Brooding
 Altered consciousness
 Rage: homicidal, suicidal
 Subsequent amnesia

Koro

Asia
Near-delusional beliefs
 Genitalia retracting
 Consequent death

Western syndromes

Multiple personality disorder
Anorexia, bulimia
Chronic fatigue syndrome (ME)

Culture is the way that different groups of people conceptualize and perceive their world and interact with their environment. It incorporates patterns of social and family relationships and religious beliefs. Cross-cultural psychiatry examines concepts of mental health and illness, their underlying causes and how symptomatology is culturally determined. It addresses issues of the universality and prevalence of psychiatric diagnoses, their treatments and their prognoses.

Concepts of symptoms, illness and healing

Our judgments concerning 'abnormal' mental symptoms or disease states frequently contain cultural assumptions of which we are unaware. The examples below are intended to make readers more critical of their own judgments.

Hallucinations and delusions of control are two of the clearest manifestations of mental illness within Western culture. In contrast, among the Xhosa of Southern Africa, hallucinations carry status.

More generally, 'possession states' (brief experiences of external control deliberately induced by ritual and/or drugs), are regarded as normal and indeed valued in most cultures.

A further example of the 'oddity' of our Western perspective is insistence on the 'mind/body' dualism. Rather than dismiss the bodily symptoms (common to many 'culture-bound' syndromes) within what we consider 'mental illness' as 'somatization', we might more appropriately regard purely 'mental' symptoms (e.g. depression, anxiety) as manifestations of Western 'psychologization'.

Cultural attitudes to death and loss are particularly important in interpreting an individual's experience of bereavement (see Chapter 8). Stages of 'normal' grieving may be very different in, for example, Great Britain, India and Greece, and cultural norms cannot be ignored in diagnosing 'abnormal' grief reactions.

The attribution of abnormal personality (see Chapter 12) is particularly dependent on cultural norms. For example, within Western countries, the 'antisocial' personality may be understandable and even have survival value in individuals from deprived inner-city areas with chronic exposure to violent crime, particularly where these are not offset by a stable family environment.

Culture may also influence attitudes to healing, a concept which is wider in non-Western societies, taking into account kinship relationships and links with the supernatural world. Elaborate rituals are often involved; the 'ward round' could be seen as a Western equivalent. Acceptance of treatment implies a shared belief in illness and in the legitimacy of intervention. For example, some Christian sects may accept conventional diagnoses but nonetheless oppose treatment as an 'artificial' intervention with God's will.

Culture and standardized diagnosis

The Kraepelinian approach to psychiatric diagnosis and classification (see Chapter 2), itself a reflection of Western culture rather than culture-independent, remains central to ICD-10 and DSM-IV-TR. It relies on the elicitation of patterns of symptoms and signs that are brought together to make 'reliable' diagnoses. The 'reliability' (or reproducibility) of such symptoms and signs is, however, questionable. The World Health Organization carried out a cross-cultural investigation of the process of psychiatric diagnosis, the International Pilot Study on Schizophrenia (IPSS), in the 1960s and 1970s. The IPSS showed that, although psychotic symptoms (delusions and hallucinations) elicited from individual patient interviews showed satisfactory reliability, clinical signs (e.g. incongruous or flat affect) were much less reliable and corroborative evidence (family, work and social background) less so still. At diagnostic level, psychotic disorders (including psychotic depression as well as schizophrenia) could be identified reliably, but neurotic and dissociative diagnoses were much less secure. It is noteworthy that many so-called 'culture-bound' syndromes have dissociative features.

As a step towards the recognition of these issues, DSM-IV-TR (although retaining multiple cultural assumptions within the axes of 'psychosocial and environmental problems' and 'global functioning') contains an 'outline' for 'cultural formulation'.

Culture and epidemiology

The IPSS established that the prevalence of schizophrenia was remarkably stable across cultures, although its prognosis was better in non-Western societies. This may reflect greater availability of home support without high expressed emotion and the absence of a stigmatizing 'label' of chronic schizophrenia. In contrast, the prevalence of depression was much more variable and its presentation in non-Western groups was often with somatic symptoms. Even for schizophrenia, cultural factors within a multicultural society may influence prevalence. For example, in the UK, an excess prevalence of schizophrenia is reported among African-Caribbeans. This may reflect several factors including misdiagnosis of affective disorders as schizophrenia; errors in estimating the total Afro-Caribbean population; cultural patterns of substance misuse (including a high prevalence of cannabis [Ganja]-induced psychoses); the complex interaction between immigration (particularly in the case of refugees/asylum seekers) and mental illness (although the excess is also apparent in 'second generation' African-Caribbeans); and mental illness being an intelligible response to disadvantage and racism. Another area of concern is the high rate of overdosing among South Asian women in Birmingham compared to White British women, which might reflect 'culture conflict' in this group. Psychiatric diagnoses have been used for political purposes such as the diagnosis of 'sluggish schizophrenia' in political dissenters in the old Communist Russia.

Pharmacological response across cultures

Racial differences in distribution of enzyme polymorphisms are reflected in, for example, increased sensitivity to alcohol (and decreased prevalence of alcohol dependence) in people of Asian origin, who also appear more susceptible to drug-induced dyskinesias. Similarly, Black Americans tend to develop higher plasma levels for given doses of tricyclic antidepressants and lithium than their White counterparts, with resultantly increased sensitivity to both therapeutic and adverse affects.

Culture-bound syndromes

According to DSM-IV, these denote locality-specific patterns of abnormal behaviour or troubling experience. *They express core cultural concerns*. Many have been described, mostly representing somatic and/or dissociative responses to stress. A few of the better known are outlined below.

Amok, described in Africa, Asia and New Guinea, is a response to humiliation involving initial brooding followed by a period of altered consciousness with uncontrollable (usually homicidal and sometimes suicidal) rage, for which the subject has no subsequent memory. Traditionally, surviving sufferers were immune from legal redress, much as the French *crime passionnel*.

Ataque de nervios occurs in Hispanic American groups, and consists of a grief reaction characterized by fluctuating conscious level (often with subsequent amnesia), crying, shouting, trembling and difficulty in moving limbs. Hyperventilation may be important in precipitating symptoms.

Latah, which occurs in Asia and North Africa, is a response to intense stress characterized by altered consciousness, hypersuggestibility and mimicry (including echolalia and echopraxia).

Koro, found mainly in Asia, involves intense anxiety centred on the belief that one's genitalia are retracting and that their disappearance will result in death. The traditional management is to tie a string around the penis and pull. Koro is associated with local tradition that ghosts have no genitals and is thus not delusional.

Brain fag is found mainly in African students, and is characterized by concentration difficulties, vague somatic complaints and depressed mood.

Some 'Western' syndromes, including multiple personality disorder, overdosing, anorexia nervosa, bulimia nervosa and chronic fatigue syndrome (myalgic encephalomyelitis [ME]) may also be considered 'culture-bound'.

Unusual psychiatric syndromes

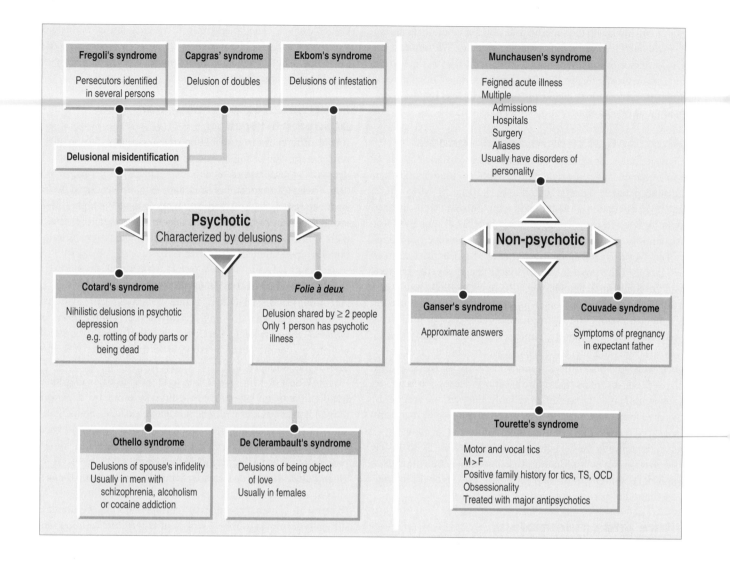

The features of the best described syndromes are summarized below, although it must be borne in mind that most have not been studied systematically. They can conveniently be divided into psychotic (characterized by delusions and hallucinations) and non-psychotic syndromes.

Psychotic
Delusional misidentification syndrome (DMS)
Several types of this syndrome have been described (*Capgras'*, *Fregoli'*, *intermetamorphosis*, *subjective doubles syndrome*), the best known are the syndromes of *Capgras* and *Fregoli*. The Capgras' syndrome was first described in 1923 by Capgras and Reboul-Lachaux and is now recognized as a psychotic state characterized by a delusion in which the patient believes that a person has been replaced by an exact double. In contrast, the rarer Fregoli's syndrome involves the delusion that the patient's persecutors are masquerading as his/her attendants (such as the doctor or nurse).

DMS may occur in schizophrenia, affective disorders and acute organic confusional states. Often an organic component accompanies these syndromes and sometimes the appearance of the syndromes heralds the development of dementia. Treatment is of the primary disorder.

Delusional parasitosis (DP)
DP is also known as Ekbom's syndrome (although the term is also used to describe a neurological syndrome of 'restless legs'). Sufferers (female/male ratio 3 : 1) believe that insects are colonizing their body, particularly the skin and eyes. Initial presentation is often to public health workers (with persistent demands for deinfestation) or to dermatologists or infectious disease physicians, with importuning and bizarre requests for investigation and treatment. Delusions may be circumscribed or part of a schizophrenic or depressive illness. Antipsychotics and/or antidepressants are the mainstay of treatment.

Folie à deux

Folie à deux consists of a delusional belief that is shared by two or more people (usually within a family), of whom only one has other psychotic features. The pair are often isolated from others in terms of distance or due to cultural or language barriers. The delusion is usually persecutory or hypochondriacal, and the psychotic individual (principal) tends to be more intelligent and better educated, and has a dominating influence over the non-psychotic (more submissive) recipient(s). Diagnosis of the principal is most commonly schizophrenia but may be an affective disorder or dementia, and primary treatment is of the underlying condition. A period of separation, followed by supportive individual and/or family therapy focused on the recipient may be helpful.

De Clerambault's syndrome (erotomania)

The patient (usually female) has the unfounded and delusional belief that someone (usually a man of higher social status) is in love with her. The patient makes inappropriate advances to the object of her passion and becomes angry (and sometimes violent) when rejected. The syndrome may exist in isolation, or as part of an affective (usually manic) disorder or, more rarely, schizophrenia. When men are affected they present a greater forensic problem. Management frequently involves hospitalization (sometimes compulsory) to prevent harassment or injury. Underlying conditions should be treated as appropriate; where none is identified neuroleptics may be useful.

Othello syndrome (OS)

OS (morbid or pathological jealousy) may complicate long-term alcohol abuse, and is also sometimes found in schizophrenia and cocaine addiction. The patient, usually male, is delusionally convinced that his spouse is being unfaithful. He goes to great lengths to produce 'evidence' of the infidelity (e.g. stains on underclothes/sheets) and to extract a confession. Paradoxically, the spouse is sometimes driven to true infidelity. There is a substantial risk of violence (even homicide); thus, distant separation may be warranted and compulsory hospitalization and treatment is often necessary. It tends to occur with a new partner.

Cotard's syndrome

Cotard's syndrome is characterized by 'nihilistic' delusions, in which the patient believes that parts of his/her body are decaying or rotting, or have ceased to exist. Patients may also believe themselves to be already dead or (paradoxically) unable to die. Although the syndrome is almost invariably found in the context of psychotic depression, the nihilistic ideas themselves often have a grandiose flavour (e.g. the world will end because of them). Electroconvulsive therapy (ECT) is usually the treatment of first choice.

Non-psychotic
Tourette's syndrome (TS)

TS was originally described by Jean Itard in 1825 but named after George Gilles de la Tourette, a French neuropsychiatrist who described nine cases in 1885 emphasizing the triad of multiple tics, echolalia and coprolalia. Current research suggests that TS occurs in 0.6–1.6% of children aged 5–18 years. Males are more often affected (3–4:1). The family history is frequently positive for tics, TS and obsessive–compulsive behaviour (OCB) obsessive–compulsive disorder (OCD). Other aetiological suggestions include pre- and perinatal difficulties and some infections. TS usually begins with facial tics such as excessive blinking; the median age at onset is 7 years. Associated features include attention-deficit hyperactivity disorder (ADHD) and OCB. Treatment is with antipsychotics (for tics), clonidine (for ADHD), selective serotonin reuptake inhibitors (SSRIs for OCB/OCD) and a behavioural approach for habit reversal (habit reversal training).

Munchausen's syndrome

Munchausen's syndrome is also known as factitious disorder and is characterized by deliberately feigned symptomatology, usually physical (e.g. abdominal pain), but can be psychiatric (e.g. hallucinations, multiple bereavements or sexual abuse). Occasionally, the disorder can be by proxy, as when a mother fakes illnesses in her child (Munchausen's syndrome by proxy [MSBP]). These result in multiple presentations to casualty departments, usually to several hospitals, with frequent admissions often culminating in surgical procedures. Patients often use multiple aliases, are often of no fixed abode and usually have no regular general practitioner (GP). When discovered, the patients usually discharge themselves against medical advice. The syndrome characteristically occurs in the setting of a severely disordered personality. Management is difficult, although confrontation without rejection may prove helpful.

Couvade syndrome

Couvade syndrome consists of the experience of symptoms resembling those of pregnancy (abdominal swelling and/or spasms, nausea and vomiting, etc.) in expectant fathers. Anxiety and psychosomatic symptoms (e.g. toothache) are common. The prevalence of mild forms is as high as 20%. The condition (which in some cultures is quite acceptable and may even be expected) is usually self-limiting and responds to counselling but often recurs in subsequent pregnancies.

Ganser's syndrome (GS)

The central feature of this syndrome is the giving of approximate, absurd and often inconsistent answers to simple questions. The patient may say 2 + 2 = 5, or, when asked the colour of snow, reply 'green'. The syndrome is also characterized by clouding of consciousness, true and/or pseudo-hallucinations (visual or auditory) and features of somatic conversion (see Chapter 25). In pure form, GS represents a dissociative reaction of defence against intolerable stress, although there may be an underlying depression warranting treatment in its own right. GS is overrepresented in prison populations. Spontaneous improvement often occurs, and is characteristically accompanied by amnesia for the abnormal behaviour. Recovery may be hastened by admission to hospital and psychotherapeutic exploration of underlying conflicts.

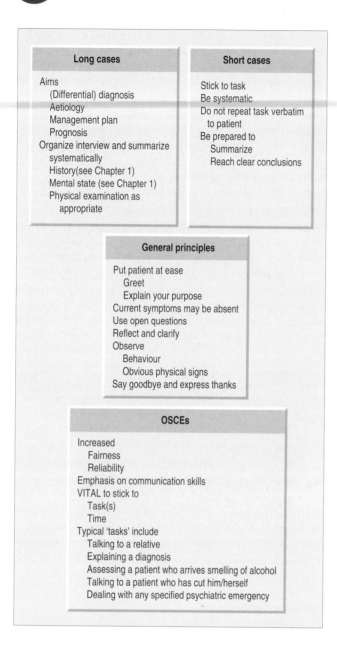

Introduction

Practice in undergraduate final examinations varies considerably between medical schools. Examiners also vary in their practice, although increasing efforts are being made to reduce such variability. Some examinations are specific to psychiatry (e.g. at the end of psychiatry placements). Psychiatry cases may also be included in more general medical examinations. The examining team may include senior doctors from a variety of specialties including general practice.

Interviewing style

Some principles remain relevant to all clinical examinations. Most patients willing and able to act as examination subjects are relatively well and may even be free of current symptoms or signs. Some patients (e.g. children, older people with cognitive impairment or people with a learning disability) may be accompanied by a relative or a professional carer. It may be useful to start by asking 'how are you?' both to make them feel you are interested in them and to get an initial gauge of their current mental state. Try wherever possible to use open rather than closed questions. 'Tell me a little more about that' is often a useful probe. Be prepared for a patient to ask you a question. It is usually best to suggest that such questions be directed at the clinical team—you are 'only' a student. Acknowledge any distress a patient shows. It is often helpful to summarize back to the patient what has been said, particularly if you are unsure what was meant. Avoid over-interpreting or extrapolating what the patient has said (not every claim of high status or profession indicates mania). Be watchful for physical signs (e.g. tremor or other extrapyramidal signs, tics, exophthalmos, evidence of liver disease, tattoos, scars, needlemarks, obviously over/underweight) and abnormal or indicative behaviours such as crying or poor eye contact.

Short cases

This part of the exam can consist of between one and four cases, depending on what cases are available on the day, how you perform and the examiner's style. You may be asked to take a particular part of the history (e.g. 'this patient has a drinking problem; please take an alcohol history') or examine a particular aspect of the mental state (e.g. 'does this patient have Schneiderian first-rank symptoms?'). You may also be asked to perform a full mental state examination or a full cognitive examination. Before you proceed with the patient, make sure you have fully understood the task(s) assigned to you. You need to greet the patient, introduce yourself and the examiner(s), explain what you have been asked to do (reiterating that this is an exam rather than a clinical situation) and be seen to put the patient at ease. It is equally important to be seen to be systematic and to give the impression that this is not the first time you have examined a psychiatric patient. Make sure you have covered all the key areas (see Chapter 1). You are likely to be asked about what you elicited and concluded when the interview has ended.

Long cases

The 'long case' involves interviewing a patient at length (usually 45–60 minutes) uninterrupted (and unobserved) with the aim of reaching a diagnosis or differential diagnosis as well as discussing aetiology, principles of medical and psychosocial management and prognosis. You will be given a few minutes after the patient has left to collect and organize your findings for the presentation. Be systematic both during the interview and the summarizing process, using headings for the history and mental state examination as outlined in Chapter 1. Clarify the patient's current status (in/outpatient, detained/informal) and any recent or significant life events (see Chapter 8). Remember that psychiatric patients often have significant physical comorbidity and that non-psychiatric examiners may be particularly interested in these aspects. Always leave enough time for a brief but appropriate physical examination. You should try and summarize the key features of the case at the end of your presentation. Try and diagnose using one or both of the classificatory systems outlined in Chapter 2. If you have had any difficulty in taking the history (some patients are suspicious or unforthcoming) it is important to say so and to remember that this should not be to your disadvantage. You may be asked to repeat some of the interview in front of the examiner(s) in which case apply the principles summarized above for short cases.

Observed structured clinical examinations (OSCEs)

These are being increasingly used to achieve greater fairness and inter-examiner reliability. From the candidate's point of view, OSCEs are very like short cases except that actors are used instead of 'real' patients and the 'tasks' are more closely structured. An OSCE examination consists of several (usually 8–12) 'stations' with a standard and relatively short time spent on each. Sticking both to task and to time are therefore vital. Communication skills are often an important element of the task, which may involve explaining something (a diagnosis, the side-effects of a drug, a prognosis) to an actor simulating a patient or a relative. Candidates may be asked to perform any relevant task within the scope of history taking or mental state examination. They can also be asked to perform tasks such as talking to a relative, explaining a diagnosis, assessing a patient who arrives smelling of alcohol, talking to a patient who has cut him/herself and discussing what to do, or dealing with any specified psychiatric emergency that a house officer may encounter. They may also be asked to assess a mental state from a video, or to write a prescription.

If, for example, you have been asked to examine cognitive function, make sure you have addressed level of consciousness, memory, orientation concentration, general knowledge and intelligence. If asked to assess suicide risk, remember to ask about mood, psychosis (including command hallucinations), past attempts and family history as well as suicidal ideation. Do not repeat the task verbatim to the patient (e.g. do not say 'I have been asked to ask you if you have any abnormal beliefs' or 'I am going to ask you about suicide'). It is also important to 'keep to task' but not to pressurize patients to give clear answers or show frustration or irritation. It can be helpful to explain to the examiners what you are doing. If you realize you have deviated from the task in hand it is better to acknowledge this and start again than to continue down the wrong road or display panic. Always thank the patient at the end of the interview, say goodbye and wish him/her well.

Further reading

Chapters 1 and 2

APA (2000) *Diagnostic and Statistical Manual of Mental Disorder*, 4th edn (revised). American Psychiatric Association, Washington, DC.

Kendell, R.E. (2001) The distinction between mental and physical illness. *British Journal of Psychiatry*, **178**, 490–493.

Sims, A. (2002) *Symptoms in the Mind*, 3rd edn. Elsevier, Amsterdam.

WHO (2002) *The ICD-10 Classification of Mental and Behavioural Disorders*. World Health Organization, Geneva.

Chapters 3 and 4

DeLisi, L.E. (1999) A critical overview of recent investigations into the genetics of schizophrenia. *Current Opinion in Psychiatry*, **12**, 29–39.

DeQuardo, J.R. (1998) Pharmacologic treatment of first-episode schizophrenia: early intervention is key to outcome. *Journal of Clinical Psychiatry*, **59** (Suppl. 19), 9–17.

McGrath, J., Saha, S., Welham, J. *et al.* (2004) A systematic review of the incidence of schizophrenia: the distribution of rates and the influence of sex, urbanicity, migrant status and methodology. *BMC Medicine*, **28** (2), 13.

Mueser, K.T. & McGurk, S.R. (2004) Schizophrenia. *Lancet*, **19**(363) (9426), 2063–2072.

NICE guidelines on schizophrenia (2002)
http://www.nice.org.uk/pdf/CG1NICEguideline.pdf

Chapter 5

Ferrier, I.N. (2001) Characterizing the ideal antidepressant therapy to achieve remission. *Journal of Clinical Psychiatry*, **62** (Suppl. 26), 10–15.

NICE guidelines on depression (2004)
http://www.nice.org.uk/pdf/CG023quickrefguide.pdf

Ronalds, C., Creed, F., Stone, K. *et al.* (1997) Outcome of anxiety and depressive disorders in primary care. *British Journal of Psychiatry*, **171**, 427–433.

Wolpert, L. (1998) *Malignant Sadness*. Faber, London.

Zisook, S., Paulus, M., Shuchter, S.R. & Judd, L.L. (1997) The many faces of depression following spousal bereavement. *Journal of Affective Disorders*, **45**, 85–94.

Chapter 6

Mitchell, P.B. & Malhi, G.S. (2004) Bipolar depression: phenomenological overview and clinical characteristics. *Bipolar Disorders*, **6**, 530–539.

Schou, M. (1998) The effect of prophylactic lithium treatment on mortality and suicidal behavior: a review for clinicians. *Journal of Affective Disorder*, **50**, 253–259.

Chapter 7

Harris, E.C. & Barraclough, B. (1997) Excess mortality of mental disorder. *British Journal of Psychiatry*, **173**, 11–53.

Hawton, K., Arensman, E., Townsend, E. *et al.* (1998) Deliberate self harm: systematic review of efficacy of psychosocial and pharmacological treatments in preventing repetition. *BMJ (Clinical Research Ed.)*, **317**, 441–447.

Hawton, K., Fagg, J., Simkin, S., Bale, E. & Bond, A. (1997) Trends in deliberate self-harm in Oxford, 1985–1995. Implications for clinical services and the prevention of suicide. *British Journal of Psychiatry*, **171**, 556–560.

Jordan, J.R. & McMenamy, J. (2004) Interventions for suicide survivors: a review of the literature. *Suicide and Life-Threatening Behaviour*, **4**, 337–349.

NICE Guidelines on self-harm (2004)
http://www.nice.org.uk/pdf/CG016NICEguideline.pdf

Chapter 8

Frueh, B.C., Buckley, T.C., Cusack, K.J. *et al.* (2004) Cognitive–behavioral treatment for PTSD among people with severe mental illness: a proposed treatment model. *Journal of Psychiatric Practice*, **10**(1), 26–38.

NICE guidelines (draft) on post-traumatic stress disorder (2004)
http://www.nice.org.uk/pdf/PTSD_2ndcons_fullguideline.pdf

Turnbull, G.J. (1998) A review of post-traumatic stress disorder. Part II: treatment. *Injury*, **260**(29), 169–175.

Yehuda, R. (1998) Psychoneuroendocrinology of post-traumatic stress disorder. *Psychiatric Clinics of North America*, **21**, 359–379.

Chapter 9

Roy-Byrne, P.P. & Wagner, A. (2004) Primary care perspectives on generalized anxiety disorder. *Journal of Clinical Psychiatry*, **65** (Suppl. 13), 20–26.

Simon, N. & Pollack, M. (1998) Current status and future prospects for anxiolytic drug therapy. *Primary Care Psychiatry*, **4**, 157–167.

Chapter 10

Greist, J.H., Bandelow, B., Hollander, E. *et al.* (2003) World Council of Anxiety (WCA) recommendations for the long-term treatment of obsessive–compulsive disorder in adults. *CNS Spectrums*, **8** (Suppl 1), 7–16.

Skoog, G. & Skoog, I. (1999) A 40-year follow-up of patients with obsessive–compulsive disorder. *Archives of General Psychiatry*, **56**, 121–127.

Chapter 11

Dare, C., Eisler, I., Russell, G., Treasure, J. & Dodge, L. (2001) Psychological therapies for adults with anorexia nervosa. RCT of outpatient treatments. *British Journal of Psychiatry* **178**, 216–221.

Gowers, S.G. & Shore, A. (2001) Development of weight and shape concerns in the aetiology of eating disorders. *British Journal of Psychiatry*, **179**, 236–242.

NICE guidelines on eating disorders (2004)
http://www.nice.org.uk/pdf/cg009niceguidance.pdf

Steiner, H. & Lock, J. (1998) Anorexia nervosa and bulimia nervosa in children and adolescents: a review of the past 10 years. *Journal of the American Academy of Child and Adolescent Psychiatry*, **37**, 352–359.

Chapter 12
Paris, J. (2004) Borderline or bipolar? Distinguishing borderline personality disorder from bipolar spectrum disorders. *Harvard Review of Psychiatry*, **12**(3), 140–145.

Tyrer, P. (1994) What are the borders of borderline personality disorder? *Acta Psychiatrica Scandinavica. Supplementum*, **379**, 38–44.

Tyrer, P., Gunderson, J., Lyons, M. & Tohen, M. (1997) Extent of comorbidity between mental state and personality disorders. *Journal of Personality Disorders*, **11**, 242–259.

Chapters 13 and 14
Department of Health (1999) *Drug Misuse and Dependence — Guidelines on Clinical Management*. HMSO, London.

Ghodse, H. (1995) *Drug and Addiction Behaviour. A Guide to Treatment*, 2nd edn. Blackwell Science, Oxford.

Tupala, E. & Tiihonen, J. (2004) Dopamine and alcoholism: neurobiological basis of ethanol abuse. *Progress in Neuro-psychopharmacology and Biological Psychiatry*, **28**(8), 1221–1247.

Chapter 15
Barry, S. (1997) Depression in pregnancy and childbirth. In: *Depression and Physical Illness* (eds M.M. Robertson & C.L.E. Katona), pp. 115–132. John Wiley and Sons, Chichester.

Connolly, M. (2001) Premenstrual syndrome: an update on definitions, diagnosis and management. *Advances in Psychiatric Treatment*, **7**(6), 469–477.

Evans, J., Heron, J., Francomb, H., Oke, S. & Golding, J. (2001) Cohort study of depressed mood during pregnancy and after childbirth. *BMJ (Clinical Research Ed.)*, **323**, 257–260.

Oates, M. (2003) Suicide: the leading cause of maternal death. *British Journal of Psychiatry*, **183**, 279–282.

Chapter 16
Baldwin, R., Graham, G., Chiu, E. & Katona, C. (2002) *Guidelines on Depression in Older people — Practising the Evidence*. Martin Dunitz, London.

Katona, C. & Livingston, G. (2002) How well do antidepressants work in older people? A systematic review of number needed to treat. *Journal of Affective Disorders*, **69**(1–3), 47–52.

Chapter 17
Macdonald, A.J.D. (1998) Delirium. In: *Geriatric Medicine and Gerontology* (eds R. Tallis, H. Fillit & J.C. Brocklehurst), 5th edn, pp. 685–699. Churchill Livingstone, Edinburgh.

Reischies, F.M. & Diefenbacher, A. (2004) Delirium in general hospital inpatients: German developments. *Advances in Psychosomatic Medicine*, **26**, 128–136.

Chapter 18
Russell, E.M. & Burns, A. (1998) Dementia: clinical presentation and management. In: *Geriatric Medicine and Gerontology* (eds R. Tallis, H. Fillit & J.C. Brocklehurst), 5th edn, pp. 727–740. Churchill Livingstone, Edinburgh.

Snowden, J.S., Neary, D. & Mann, D.M.A. (2002) Frontotemporal dementia. *British Journal of Psychiatry*, **180**, 140–143.

Stewart, R. (2002) Vascular dementia: a diagnosis running out of time. *British Journal of Psychiatry*, **180**, 152–156.

Chapters 19 and 20
Frumin, M., Chisholm, T., Dickey, C.C. & Daffner, K.R. (1998) Psychiatric and behavioral problems. *Neurologic Clinics*, **16**, 521–544.

Obeso, J.A., Rodríguez-Oroz, M.C., Rodríguez, M., Arbizu, T. & Gimenéz-Amaya, J.M. (1997) Basal ganglia pathophysiology: a critical review. *Advances in Neurology*, **74**, 3–18.

Ring, H.A. & Serra-Mestres, J. (2002) Neuropsychiatry of the basal ganglia. *Journal of Neurology, Neurosurgery, and Psychiatry*, **72**(1), 12–21.

Sanders, R.D. & Keshavan, M.S. (1998) The neurologic examination in adult psychiatry: from soft signs to hard science. *Journal of Neuropsychiatry and Clinical Neurosciences*, **230**, 395–404.

Chapters 21 and 22
Cassidy, L.J. & Jellinek, M.S. (1998) Approaches to recognition and management of childhood psychiatric disorders in pediatric primary care. *Pediatric Clinics of North America*, **45**, 1037–1052.

Courtney, D.B. (2004) Selective serotonin reuptake inhibitor and venlafaxine use in children and adolescents with major depressive disorder: a systematic review of published randomized controlled trials. *Canadian Journal of Psychiatry*, **49**(8), 557–563.

Chapter 23
Berenson, C.K. (1998) Frequently missed diagnoses in adolescent psychiatry. *Psychiatric Clinics of North America*, **21**, 917–926.

Worrall, A., O'Herlihy, A., Banerjee, S. *et al.* (2004) Inappropriate admission of young people with mental disorder to adult psychiatric wards and paediatric wards: cross sectional study of 6 months' activity. *BMJ (Clinical Research Ed.)*, **10** (328), 867.

Chapter 24
Hassiotis, A. & Hall, I. (2004) Behavioural and cognitive–behavioural interventions for outwardly-directed aggressive behaviour in people with learning disabilities. *Cochrane Database of Systematic Reviews (Online)*, **18**(4), CD003406.

Russell, O. (ed.) (1997) *Seminars in the Psychiatry of Learning Disabilities*. Royal College of Psychiatrists and Gaskell Press, London.

Chapter 25
Antonowicz, J.L. (1998) Missed diagnoses in consultation liaison psychiatry. *Psychiatric Clinics of North America*, **21**(3), 705–714.

Arolt, V. & Rothermundt, M. (2004) Depression in medical patients. *Advances in Psychosomatic Medicine*, **26**, 98–117.

Gjaerum, B. & Blomhoff, S. (1998) Assessment of the mental state in medically ill adults. *Current Opinion in Psychiatry*, **11**, 643–647.

Chapter 26

Burns, T. & Bristow, M. (1997) The role of the GP in the management of schizophrenia. *Primary Care Psychiatry*, **3**, 169–173.

Shiels, C., Gabbay, M., Dowrick, C. & Hulbert, C. (2004) Depression in men attending a rural general practice: factors associated with prevalence of depressive symptoms and diagnosis. *British Journal of Psychiatry*, **185**, 239–244.

Thornicroft, G., Wykes, T., Holloway, F., Johnson, S. & Szmukler, G. (1998) From efficacy to effectiveness in community mental health services. PRiSM psychosis study 10. *British Journal of Psychiatry*, **173**, 423–427.

Chapter 27

Coid, J.W. (2002) Personality disorders in prisoners and their motivation for dangerous and disruptive behaviour. *Criminal Behaviour and Mental Health*, **12**(3), 209–226.

Exworthy, T. (1998) Institutions and services in forensic psychiatry. *Journal of Forensic Psychiatry*, **9**, 395–412.

Taylor, P.J. & Gunn, J. (1999) Homicides by people with mental illness: myth and reality. *British Journal of Psychiatry*, **174**, 9–14.

Chapter 28

Jones, R. (ed.) (1994) *Mental Health Act Manual*. Sweet & Maxwell, London.

Mental Health Bill (draft) http://www.dh.gov.uk/PublicationsAndStatistics/Publications/PublicationsLegislation/PublicationsLegislationArticle/fs/en?CONTENT_ID=4088910&chk=6GB8PU

Chapter 29

Royal College of Psychiatrists (1998) *The Management of Imminent Violence*. Gaskell Press, London.

Chapter 30

Leiblum, S.R. (1998) Definition and classification of female sexual disorders. *International Journal of Impotence Research*, **10** (Suppl. 2), S104–S106.

Wylie, K. (2004) Gender related disorders. *BMJ (Clinical Research Ed.)*, **11** (329), 615–617.

Chapter 31

Pajonk, F.G. & Naber, D. (1998) Human immunodeficiency virus and mental disorders. *Current Opinion in Psychiatry*, **11**, 305–310.

Price, S. & Goyette, J. (2003) Role of the psychiatrist in the care of patients with hepatitis C and HIV/AIDS. *Psychiatric Quarterly*, **74**(3), 261–276.

Chapter 32

Robins, C.J. & Chapman, A.L. (2004) Dialectical behavior therapy: current status, recent developments, and future directions. *Journal of Personality Disorders*, **18**(1), 73–89.

Salkovskis, P.M., Forrester, E. & Richards, C. (1998) Cognitive–behavioural approach to understanding obsessional thinking. *British Journal of Psychiatry*, **173** (Suppl. 35), 53–63.

Chapters 33 and 34

Cookson, J., Taylor, D. & Katona, C. (2003) *Drugs in Psychiatry*. Gaskell Press, London.

Cooper, S.J. & Ingram, R. (1998) Electroconvulsive therapy in current psychiatric practice. *Primary Care Psychiatry*, **4**, 169–178.

Fleischhacker, W. (1999) The psychopharmacology of schizophrenia. *Current Opinion in Psychiatry*, **103**(12), 53–59.

George, M.S. (2000) New methods of brain stimulation (ECT, MST, TMS, VNS and DBS) are improving OCD research and therapy (from the 4th IOCDC Plenary Lecture). *CNS Spectrums*, **5**, 12–17.

Nemeroff, C.B. (1998) Psychopharmacology of affective disorders in the 21st century. *Biological Psychiatry*, **44**, 515–517.

Chapter 35

Bhugra, D. & Bhui, K. (2001) African-Caribbeans and schizophrenia: contributing factors. *Advances in Psychiatric Treatment*, **7**(4), 283–291.

Cheng, A.T.A. (2001) Case definition and culture: are people all the same? *British Journal of Psychiatry*, **179**, 1–4.

Leavey, G. (2001) Too close for comfort: mental illness and the Irish in Britain. In: *Colonialism and Psychiatry* (eds D. Bhugra & R. Littlewood), pp. 167–185. Oxford University Press, Oxford.

Littlewood, R. & Lipsedge, M. (1997) *Aliens and Alienists: Ethnic Minorities and Psychiatry*, 3rd edn. Routledge, London.

Sumathipala, A., Siribaddana, S.H. & Bhugra, D. (2004) Culture-bound syndromes: the story of dhat syndrome. *British Journal of Psychiatry*, **184**, 200–210.

Chapter 36

Asher, R. (1951) Munchausen's syndrome. *Lancet*, **i**, 339–341.

Enoch, M.D. & Trethowan, W. (1991) *Uncommon Psychiatric Syndromes*. Butterworth Heinemann, Oxford.

Robertson, M.M. (2000) Tourette syndrome, associated conditions and the complexities of treatment. *Brain*, **123** (Pt 3), 425–462.

Questions

The following multiple choice questions are intended to help readers check their understanding of the material covered in the book and to aid revision. They are arranged by subject matter and their sequence corresponds with that of the chapters to which they refer.

1 Important factors to be considered in assessing a patient's speech include:
   (a) Rate
   (b) Pressure
   (c) Tone
   (d) Coherence
   (e) Perspicacity

2 Abnormal beliefs include:
   (a) Obsessions
   (b) Phobias
   (c) Ideas of reference
   (d) Autochthonous delusions
   (e) Depersonalization

3 Main ways of classifying mental disorders include:
   (a) Categorical
   (b) Dimensional
   (c) Multiaxial
   (d) Symptomatic
   (e) Pragmatic

4 ICD-10:
   (a) Uses operational definitions
   (b) Is reliant on clinical description
   (c) Measures personality disorders on axis II
   (d) Excludes organic disorders
   (e) Is published by the World Health Organization

5 Schneider's first-rank symptoms of schizophrenia include:
   (a) Thought echo
   (b) Thought block
   (c) Delusional perception
   (d) Olfactory hallucinations
   (e) Somatic passivity

6 Abnormal family processes implicated in schizophrenia include:
   (a) Oversubmissive mother
   (b) Low expressed emotion
   (c) Ambivalence
   (d) Early parental separation
   (e) Adverse life events

7 Factors predictive of a good prognosis in schizophrenia include:
   (a) Insidious onset
   (b) A strong affective component
   (c) Older age at onset
   (d) Predominantly 'positive' symptoms
   (e) Positive family history

   (f) Birth trauma
   (g) Male gender

8 The cluster of clinical features of schizophrenia described by Bleuler includes:
   (a) Affective incongruity
   (b) Ambivalence
   (c) Anhedonia
   (d) Agitation
   (e) Autochthonous delusions

9 Psychosocial factors implicated in the aetiology of depression include:
   (a) Unemployment
   (b) Being an only child
   (c) Overstimulation
   (d) Childhood abuse
   (e) High serotonin levels

10 Recognized depressive subtypes include:
   (a) Catatonic
   (b) Dysthymic
   (c) Bipolar
   (d) Atypical
   (e) Borderline

11 Mania:
   (a) Has a recurrence rate of about 20% in 10 years
   (b) Is characterized by irritability
   (c) Is associated with first-rank symptoms in 25% of cases
   (d) Is characterized by nihilistic delusions
   (e) May be treated with phenobarbitone

12 The following statements about the epidemiology of mania are true:
   (a) The typical age of onset is in the mid-teens
   (b) Lifetime risk is about 5%
   (c) It is commoner in women
   (d) It is commoner in higher socio-economic groups
   (e) Incidence is about 20/100 000 per year

13 Factors associated with a markedly increased risk of suicide include:
   (a) Drug abuse
   (b) Generalized anxiety
   (c) Unemployment
   (d) Availability of firearms
   (e) House move

14 Factors associated with a markedly increased risk of deliberate self-harm include:
   (a) Male gender
   (b) Lower socio-economic class
   (c) Living with a partner
   (d) Personality disorder
   (e) Age > 50 years

15 Features indicative of atypical grief include:
   (a) Early onset
   (b) Rapid progression

(c) Despair

(d) Guilt

(e) Shock

16 Post-traumatic stress disorder:
   (a) Is usually associated with anxiety symptoms
   (b) More frequently occurs following natural than 'man-made' disasters
   (c) Is always self-limiting
   (d) Responds well to benzodiazepines
   (e) Can be treated with trauma-focussed cognitive–behaviour therapy (CBT)

17 Characteristic clinical features of generalized anxiety disorder include:
   (a) Apprehensive expectations
   (b) Hypovigilance
   (c) Fear of going crazy
   (d) Muscle tension
   (e) Autonomic arousal

18 Recognized treatments of anxiety disorders include:
   (a) Cognitive–behaviour therapy (CBT)
   (b) Monoamine oxidase inhibitors (MAOIs)
   (c) Maintenance benzodiazepines
   (d) Carbamazepine
   (e) Interpersonal psychotherapy (IPT)

19 Social anxiety disorders:
   (a) Occur more in males
   (b) Have an adult onset
   (c) Should be treated with antipsychotics
   (d) Respond to behavioural techniques
   (e) Can present with vomiting

20 The following is true about obsessive–compulsive disorder (OCD):
   (a) It occurs more frequently in women
   (b) It is characterized by delusions of contamination
   (c) It is associated with dopaminergic underactivity
   (d) It responds well to psychoanalysis
   (e) The lifetime risk is 10%
   (f) May be treated with deep brain stimulation

21 Bulimia nervosa:
   (a) Is characterized by carbohydrate starvation
   (b) Occurs with a female/male ratio of 3 : 1
   (c) Carries a better prognosis if the patient is underweight
   (d) May be associated with transient trance-like states
   (e) Is characterized by the presence of lanugo hair

22 Anorexia nervosa:
   (a) Carries a 10% risk of suicide
   (b) Is associated with tachycardia
   (c) Often presents in the early teenage years
   (d) Is seldom associated with binge eating
   (e) May cause life-threatening hypokalaemia
   (f) May be treated using interpersonal psychotherapy

23 The following statements about borderline personality disorder are true:
   (a) It may be known as anankastic personality disorder
   (b) Binge eating sometimes occurs
   (c) Hallucinations may be present

(d) Sufferers usually show little interest in sex

(e) Response to antidepressants is sometimes good

(f) May be treated with dialectical behaviour therapy

24 Established treatments of personality disorders include:
   (a) Dynamic psychotherapy
   (b) Therapeutic community
   (c) Limit setting
   (d) Methylphenidate
   (e) Electroconvulsive therapy (ECT)

25 Cardinal features of drug dependence include:
   (a) Intolerance
   (b) Reduced social activity
   (c) Neglect of other interests
   (d) Hallucinations
   (e) Somatic passivity

26 Physical features of opiate withdrawal include:
   (a) Mydriasis
   (b) Tremor
   (c) Diarrhoea
   (d) Piloerection
   (e) Bradycardia

27 Management of substance misuse includes:
   (a) Harm reduction
   (b) Atomoxetine
   (c) Habit reversal training
   (d) Long-term lofexidine
   (e) Maintenance benzodiazepines

28 Alcohol dependence:
   (a) Is frequently associated with a microcytic anaemia
   (b) Is frequently associated with an elevated γ-glutamyl transferase level
   (c) Is associated with atrophy of Wernicke's area
   (d) May be treated by group psychotherapy
   (e) Carries an increased risk of complex partial seizures
   (f) May be detected using the slow screen

29 Management of alcohol withdrawal includes:
   (a) Chlorpromazine to reduce risk of seizures
   (b) Ascorbic acid supplementation
   (c) Frequent changes of nursing staff
   (d) Disulfiram
   (e) Cognitive–behaviour therapy (CBT)

30 Postpartum psychosis:
   (a) Occurs after 1% of deliveries
   (b) Is usually affective
   (c) Mandates cessation of breastfeeding
   (d) Occurs more frequently following instrumental delivery
   (e) Seldom responds to electroconvulsive therapy (ECT)

31 Bonding failure:
   (a) Is more common in girls
   (b) Is associated with Tourette's syndrome
   (c) Responds to behavioural programmes
   (d) May be associated with hostility towards the baby
   (e) Is usually associated with schizophrenia

32 Non-psychotic depression after childbirth:
  (a) Usually presents within the first postpartum week
  (b) Is seldom associated with suicidal intent
  (c) Is usually inherited
  (d) Is associated with a history of premenstrual tension
  (e) Can be treated with antidepressants

33 Depression in old age:
  (a) Carries a low risk of suicide
  (b) Often presents with somatic symptoms
  (c) May present as a dementia
  (d) Seldom responds to electroconvulsive therapy (ECT)
  (e) Is more often associated with anxiety symptoms than depression earlier in life

34 The following statements concerning mania in old age are true:
  (a) It occurs more frequently in women
  (b) It may be associated with prominent subjective confusion
  (c) Elation occurs less frequently than in younger people
  (d) It may be precipitated by stroke
  (e) Response to lithium is poor

35 Characteristic clinical features of delirium include:
  (a) Confusion worst at night
  (b) Apathy
  (c) Illusions
  (d) Consistent cognitive deficits
  (e) Hypervigilance

36 Features of delirium that help distinguish it from dementia include:
  (a) Insidious onset
  (b) Presence of delusions
  (c) Tactile hallucinations
  (d) Clouding of consciousness
  (e) Flight of ideas

37 Conditions which may be mistaken for dementia include:
  (a) Normal ageing
  (b) Depression
  (c) Myxoedema
  (d) Othello syndrome
  (e) Delirium

38 The following statements concerning Alzheimer's disease are true:
  (a) Periventricular lucencies are often found on computed tomography (CT) scan
  (b) Dopaminergic neurotransmission is markedly reduced
  (c) Risk is increased in people homozygous for the E4 allele of the apolipoprotein gene
  (d) Hypertension is common
  (e) Sleep is often disrupted
  (f) A clear distinction from vascular dementia can usually be made

39 Huntington's disease:
  (a) Is associated with decreased GABAergic neurotransmission
  (b) Has autosomal recessive inheritance
  (c) The determining gene is localized on chromosome 4
  (d) Carries a 25% risk of dementia
  (e) Is associated with nucleus accumbens degeneration

40 Psychiatric complications of Parkinson's disease include:
  (a) Frontal impairment
  (b) Iatrogenic psychosis
  (c) Depression
  (d) Korsakoff's syndrome
  (e) Obsessions

41 The following statements are true about epilepsy:
  (a) Treatment with phenobarbitone may cause depression
  (b) Schizophreniform psychoses are associated with a left-sided temporal seizure focus
  (c) Mania is common
  (d) Risk of suicide is increased most markedly in absence seizures
  (e) Pseudo-seizures may be associated with high prolactin levels
  (f) Depression occurs in 50%

42 Hypothyroidism may present as:
  (a) Asperger's syndrome
  (b) Dementia
  (c) Depression
  (d) Anxiety
  (e) Anorexia

43 The following features of truancy help to distinguish it from school refusal:
  (a) The whereabouts of the child during school hours are not known
  (b) Anxiety symptoms are prominent
  (c) Comorbid conduct disorder
  (d) Good academic performance
  (e) Cyclothymic personality

44 The following statements about child abuse are true:
  (a) The presentation may be of Munchausen's syndrome by proxy
  (b) Victims are usually of low birthweight
  (c) There is frequently a history of early maternal separation
  (d) Abusing parents have themselves often been abused
  (e) Social Class I is overrepresented

45 Attention-deficit hyperactivity disorder (ADHD) in childhood:
  (a) Is commoner in boys
  (b) Is characterized by grandiosity
  (c) May be treated with dexamphetamine
  (d) Seldom persists into adult life
  (e) May be predictive of adult antisocial personality disorder

46 Clinical features of autism include:
  (a) Impaired language development
  (b) Hemiparesis
  (c) Ritualistic behaviours
  (d) Auditory hallucinations
  (e) Aloofness

47 Conduct disorder in adolescence:
  (a) Often coexists with substance abuse
  (b) Is seldom associated with criminal behaviour
  (c) Is more common in females
  (d) May respond to family therapy
  (e) Is often associated with depressive symptoms

48 The following statements are true about schizophrenia in adolescence:
   (a) Onset is commonly before the age of 15 years
   (b) The presentation may be with deteriorating school performance
   (c) Social withdrawal is rare
   (d) Schneiderian first-rank symptoms may be fleeting
   (e) Extrapyramidal reactions to neuroleptics are rare

49 Characteristic features of Down syndrome include:
   (a) High arched feet
   (b) Cardiac septal defects
   (c) Multiple palmar creases
   (d) Hyperthyroidism
   (e) Flat occiput

50 Common psychiatric complications of learning disability include:
   (a) Conversion symptoms
   (b) Hallucinations
   (c) Phobic anxiety
   (d) Depressed mood
   (e) Primary delusional perception

51 Testamentary capacity requires:
   (a) IQ > 90
   (b) Understanding the value of one's property
   (c) Understanding what a will is
   (d) The absence of mental illness
   (e) Understanding who might have a legitimate claim on one's property

52 Symptoms triggering referral of medical patients for psychiatric opinion include:
   (a) Chronic pain
   (b) Fatigue
   (c) Agitation
   (d) Confusion
   (e) Aggressivity

53 Depression in a physically ill patient frequently presents with:
   (a) Suicidal threats
   (b) Guilt
   (c) Fatigue
   (d) Requests for antidepressants
   (e) Prominent anxiety symptoms

54 Common psychiatric disorders as seen in primary care:
   (a) Occur in 50% of women within a year
   (b) Seldom respond to counselling
   (c) Should always be referred to a psychiatrist
   (d) Often present with physical symptoms
   (e) Usually have a florid presentation

55 Community care of patients with severe psychiatric illness:
   (a) Is cheaper than institutional care
   (b) Requires detailed care planning
   (c) Is formalized in the 1987 Care in the Community Act
   (d) Has to be based in community mental health centres
   (e) Can prevent institutionalization

56 Fitness to plead requires:
   (a) Literacy
   (b) Understanding of the nature of the charges being faced
   (c) Capacity to instruct counsel

   (d) The absence of current psychotic features
   (e) Understanding of the meaning of a guilty plea

57 Significant associations between crime and mental illness include:
   (a) Depression and shoplifting
   (b) Depression and fraud
   (c) Dementia and sexual offences
   (d) Learning disability and arson
   (e) Alcohol dependence and driving offences

58 The following statements concerning the 1983 Mental Health Act (England and Wales) are true:
   (a) Section 2 lasts for up to 6 months
   (b) Section 41 restricted patients may not be discharged without the Prime Minister's consent
   (c) Consent to electroconvulsive therapy (ECT) is covered in Section 58
   (d) Patients on Section 3 can only go on leave with the written consent of the Responsible Medical Officer
   (e) Mental illness is not defined within the Act

59 Compulsory admission under the 1983 Mental Health Act (England and Wales) requires:
   (a) Current mental illness
   (b) Dangerousness
   (c) Refusal of voluntary admission or treatment
   (d) The presence of the patient's general practitioner (GP)
   (e) Application by a social worker

60 Risk assessment:
   (a) Should include urgent full physical examination
   (b) Does not require respect for patient confidentiality
   (c) Should be fully documented in care notes
   (d) Should take note of command hallucinations
   (e) Requires attention to family history

61 Common sexual dysfunctions in men include:
   (a) Lack of sexual enjoyment
   (b) Ejaculatory failure
   (c) Pain on intercourse
   (d) Fetishism
   (e) Transsexuality

62 Variations of the sexual act include:
   (a) Exhibitionism
   (b) Paedophilia
   (c) Frotteurism
   (d) Necrophilia
   (e) Dyspareunia

63 The following statements about human immunodeficiency virus (HIV) are true:
   (a) The world-wide death toll is approximately 5 million
   (b) Acute stress reactions are common
   (c) Self-help groups can play an important role
   (d) Azidothymidine (AZT) can induce schizophrenia
   (e) Parietal hypoperfusion is characteristic of HIV-I associated neuropsychiatric dysfunction

64 Psychoanalysis:
   (a) Stresses the importance of childhood experience
   (b) Is indicated in bipolar disorders
   (c) Requires the ability to cope with painful insights
   (d) Was introduced by Carl Jung
   (e) Relies on countertransference

65 Interpersonal psychotherapy (IPT):
   (a) Was devised by Sigmund Freud
   (b) Is indicated for psychotic depression
   (c) Has role transition as a focus
   (d) Is useful in eating disorders
   (e) Links interpersonal difficulties with severity of depression

66 Phenothiazines:
   (a) Block cholinergic receptors
   (b) Cause menorrhagia
   (c) Are excreted intact in the urine
   (d) Seldom cause tardive dyskinesia
   (e) Are associated with haemolytic jaundice

67 Selective serotonin reuptake inhibitors (SSRIs):
   (a) Are only indicated in the treatment of depressive disorders
   (b) Are usually given by injection
   (c) Achieve a response rate of 90% in clinical practice
   (d) Often cause headache
   (e) Often cause dry mouth
   (f) Are indicated for depression in children

68 Indications for electroconvulsive therapy (ECT) include:
   (a) Cotard's syndrome
   (b) Catatonia
   (c) Anxiety
   (d) Puerperal psychosis
   (e) Fregoli's syndrome

69 Side-effects of lithium include:
   (a) Oedema
   (b) Hyperthyroidism
   (c) Diarrhoea
   (d) Fine tremor
   (e) Leucopenia

70 Benzodiazepines:
   (a) Should not be given to people with epilepsy
   (b) May induce tolerance
   (c) Inhibit the excitatory effects of GABA
   (d) Are indicated in the treatment of alcohol withdrawal
   (e) Potentiate alcohol

71 The following statements about cross-cultural syndromes are true:
   (a) Amok is a response to humiliation
   (b) Echopraxia is a central feature of Koro
   (c) Dissociative features are frequently found
   (d) Latah is frequently found in South America
   (e) Hyperventilation may precipitate 'ataque de nervios'

72 Tourette's syndrome:
   (a) Is characterized by multiple tics
   (b) Responds well to benzodiazepines
   (c) More often affects men than women
   (d) Is associated with early maternal separation
   (e) Usually presents in early adult life

73 The following statements about unusual psychiatric syndromes are true:
   (a) De Clerambault's syndrome may be a feature of mania
   (b) The main risk in Othello syndrome is of suicide
   (c) Delusional parasitosis was first described by Ganser
   (d) Couvade syndrome is a form of delusional misidentification
   (e) In *folie à deux* both victims have a psychotic illness

Answers

1 (a) true, (b) true, (c) true, (d) true, (e) false

2 (a) false, (b) false, (c) true, (d) true, (e) false

3 (a) true, (b) true, (c) true, (d) false, (e) false

4 (a) false, (b) true, (c) false, (d) false, (e) true

5 (a) true, (b) false, (c) true, (d) false, (e) true

6 (a) false, (b) false, (c) false, (d) false, (e) false

7 (a) false, (b) true, (c) true, (d) true, (e) false, (f) true, (g) false

8 (a) true, (b) true, (c) false, (d) false, (e) false

9 (a) true, (b) false, (c) false, (d) true, (e) false

10 (a) false, (b) true, (c) true, (d) true, (e) false

11 (a) false, (b) true, (c) false, (d) false, (e) false

12 (a) true, (b) false, (c) true, (d) true, (e) true

13 (a) true, (b) false, (c) true, (d) true, (e) true

14 (a) false, (b) true, (c) false, (d) true, (e) false

15 (a) false, (b) false, (c) true, (d) true, (e) false

16 (a) true, (b) false, (c) false, (d) false, (e) true

17 (a) true, (b) false, (c) false, (d) true, (e) true

18 (a) true, (b) true, (c) false, (d) false, (e) false

19 (a) false, (b) true, (c) false, (d) true, (e) true

20 (a) false, (b) false, (c) false, (d) false, (e) false, (f) true

21 (a) false, (b) false, (c) false, (d) true, (e) false

22 (a) false, (b) true, (c) true, (d) false, (e) true, (f) true

23 (a) false, (b) true, (c) true, (d) false, (e) true, (f) true

24 (a) true, (b) true, (c) true, (d) false, (e) false

25 (a) false, (b) true, (c) true, (d) false, (e) false

26 (a) false, (b) true, (c) true, (d) true, (e) false

27 (a) true, (b) false, (c) false, (d) true, (e) false

28 (a) false, (b) true, (c) false, (d) true, (e) false, (f) true

29 (a) false, (b) false, (c) false, (d) false, (e) false

30 (a) false, (b) true, (c) false, (d) true, (e) false

31 (a) false, (b) false, (c) true, (d) true, (e) false

32 (a) false, (b) true, (c) false, (d) true, (e) true

33 (a) false, (b) true, (c) true, (d) false, (e) true

34 (a) true, (b) true, (c) true, (d) true, (e) false

35 (a) true, (b) true, (c) true, (d) false, (e) true

36 (a) false, (b) false, (c) true, (d) true, (e) false

37 (a) true, (b) true, (c) true, (d) false, (e) true

38 (a) false, (b) false, (c) true, (d) false, (e) true, (f) false

39 (a) true, (b) false, (c) true, (d) false, (e) false

40 (a) true, (b) true, (c) true, (d) false, (e) true

41 (a) true, (b) true, (c) false, (d) false, (e) false, (f) false

42 (a) false, (b) true, (c) true, (d) true, (e) false

43 (a) true, (b) false, (c) true, (d) false, (e) false

44 (a) true, (b) true, (c) true, (d) true, (e) false

45 (a) true, (b) false, (c) true, (d) false, (e) true

46 (a) true, (b) false, (c) true, (d) false, (e) true

47 (a) true, (b) false, (c) false, (d) true, (e) true

48 (a) false, (b) true, (c) false, (d) true, (e) false

49 (a) false, (b) true, (c) false, (d) false, (e) true

50 (a) true, (b) true, (c) true, (d) true, (e) false

51 (a) false, (b) true, (c) true, (d) false, (e) true

52 (a) true, (b) true, (c) true, (d) true, (e) true

53 (a) true, (b) false, (c) true, (d) false, (e) true

54 (a) false, (b) false, (c) false, (d) true, (e) false

55 (a) false, (b) true, (c) false, (d) false, (e) true

56 (a) false, (b) true, (c) true, (d) false, (e) true

57 (a) true, (b) false, (c) true, (d) true, (e) true

58 (a) false, (b) false, (c) true, (d) true, (e) true

59 (a) false, (b) false, (c) true, (d) false, (e) false

60 (a) false, (b) false, (c) true, (d) true, (e) false

61 (a) false, (b) true, (c) false, (d) false, (e) true

62 (a) true, (b) false, (c) true, (d) false, (e) false

63 (a) false, (b) true, (c) true, (d) false, (e) false

64 (a) true, (b) false, (c) true, (d) false, (e) false

65 (a) false, (b) false, (c) true, (d) true, (e) true

66 (a) true, (b) false, (c) false, (d) false, (e) false

67 (a) false, (b) false, (c) false, (d) true, (e) false, (f) false

68 (a) true, (b) true, (c) false, (d) true, (e) false

69 (a) true, (b) false, (c) true, (d) true, (e) false

70 (a) false, (b) true, (c) false, (d) true, (e) true

71 (a) true, (b) false, (c) true, (d) false, (e) true

72 (a) true, (b) false, (c) true, (d) false, (e) false

73 (a) true, (b) false, (c) false, (d) false, (e) false

Index

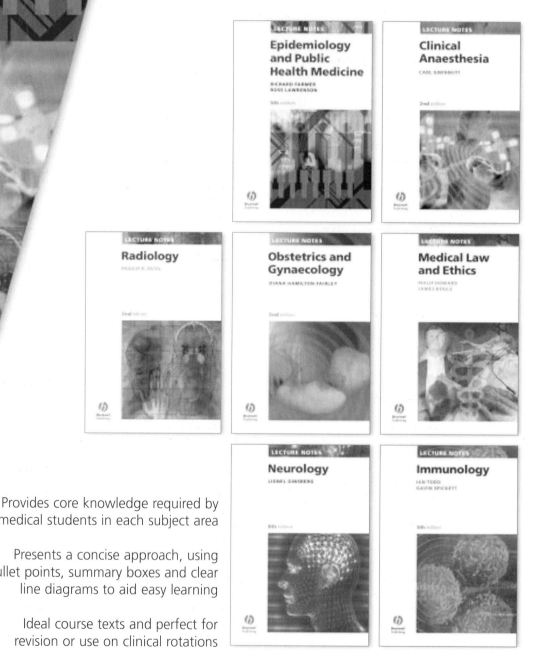